DID YOU KNOW . . .

—that overeating can be caused by foods that *make* you hungry?

—that diet pills can cause psychosis?

—that what you eat can help you resist poisoning from toxic metals in the air?

—how nutrition can help cure alcoholism?

Not "just another" slimming book, BE SLIM *AND* HEALTHY combines a simple, *natural* method for healthy slimming with fascinating information on why this program works so well and just what it means to your whole body.

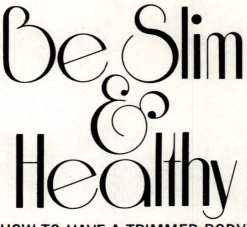

Be Slim & Healthy

HOW TO HAVE A TRIMMER BODY THE NATURAL WAY

LINDA A. CLARK, M.A.

Keats Publishing, Inc.   New Canaan, Connecticut

BE SLIM AND HEALTHY

Pivot Edition published 1972

Library of Congress Catalogue Card Number: 72-83520

PIVOT ORIGINAL HEALTH BOOKS are published by Keats Publishing, Inc., 212 Elm Street, New Canaan, Connecticut 06840

Contents

Be Slim & Healthy

CHAPTER 1

The Real Reason Why You Are Overweight

The guests at the party looked like peas in a pod. Most of the men were slightly pasty-faced, with thinning hair and a paunch. They were gulping down their cocktails and reaching out for more hors d'oeuvres. There was a startling similarity among the women present; their hair had been faultlessly set at a beauty salon; their nails perfectly manicured. They were fashionably dressed, slim as reeds, and heavily made up. At first glance, they appeared to be "well preserved" until you looked closer. Behind the facade, something alarming became apparent.

Almost every woman had dry skin and straw-like, lustreless hair, even though the beauty operator had tried to hide this with conditioners and sprays. Even worse, on closer inspection, they looked discontented, nervous and trying to appear frantically gay for the benefit of their audience. Each sipped her drink daintily and looked hungrily at the hors d'oeuvre tray, fighting the temptation to eat the whole lot. It was apparent that these women were dieting. They looked sylph-like, but it was clearly evident that underneath they felt like wrecks. They pretended to be enjoying themselves, but once they were outside the host's door, they probably gave vent to their long pent-up ill humor and irritation, common by-products of a reducing diet.

This picture, as you know, is reproduced thousands of times in every hamlet and city in America. Overweight is a national—even an international—epidemic. It is a disease caused by a condition *which is preventable and*

1

controllable, and this unique approach, to my knowledge, has not been discussed in any book prior to this one. When you see the real reason for overweight, you will say, "How simple! Why hadn't I ever thought of that before?" There is a simple explanation for the prevention and control of overweight.

Another and Another

Let me assure you I am not offering you one more palliative. There have already been too many. The other day I picked up a copy of a popular woman's magazine. On the cover were large red headlines: NEW DIET BY A DOCTOR HELPS YOU LOSE ELEVEN POUNDS IN ONE WEEK! Women were lining up to buy the magazine, hoping that perhaps *this* diet, *this* time, would work. Such articles are gold mines for magazine publishers, but they are just another disappointment to the poor would-be reducer. Why? Because the real cause has not even been guessed or touched upon. There are thousands upon thousands of reducing diets, but after a few weeks, and the loss of a few pounds, the reducer can't stick with it any longer. She becomes ravenous *and* nervous until finally she can stand it no longer; the minute her family has left the house, she shuts the front door and opens the refrigerator door. She starts stuffing herself until she is no longer hungry and no longer a convert to *that* diet. As the pounds pile up again, within a few weeks she is trying another. But, meanwhile the interludes are blissful for her, and her family, who have been scapegoats for the case of nerves they have been forced to endure from a miserable, irritable, unhappy dieter. Is it really worth it?

Being thin these days is an image all women seem to try to attain. And some of them don't even need to reduce; they just want to keep up with their friends. Reducing becomes an obsession. Many women try to look like the too-thin models in the chic fashion magazine. Unlike those people who are compulsive eaters, others are obsessed by compulsive reducing, the opposite extreme. These unfortunates weigh daily, and if they gain a pound or less (weight can fluctuate temporarily in either direction without being serious), these women panic. I know three of them. They can think of little else. They feel guilt-ridden when they eat. Such people can make themselves and their families miserable.

If you can't get into a dress you wore 20 years ago because you have changed an inch or so in your measurements, forget it! Childbirth, even improved nutrition, can make some changes in your dimensions and this may be a sign you are either normal for your age, or even better than you were 20 years ago.

Salvator Cutolo, M.D., believes that many people should not be thin. He feels it is better to be a little overweight, even up to 10 pounds. Although excessive weight is to be discouraged for both health and appearance reasons, Dr. Cutolo believes that a small surplus of weight gives you a reserve of energy if you should need it. Women who are emaciated or too thin are more nervous and harder to live with. I am sure both husbands and families would prefer wives and mothers to be five pounds overweight and be cheerful and relaxed, rather than to make a fetish of being thin and snap at their families or feel irritable due to a reducing obsession. Life is too short. Decide which is more important.

The time may come when being slightly overweight will be just as fashionable as being over-thin is today. Why? Look at a woman who is not scrawny. Her skin is plump and smooth, like that of a girl. She is cheerful. Her hair has more sheen, her eyes more shine, and her nerves are covered by a bit of padding; they are not raw. Any man will tell you she is more lovable and cuddlesome. As she is more relaxed, so is her family. In short, she *feels* better and thus with more energy and sparkle, she *looks* better. And, don't forget that following the reducing cult can also cause premature aging.

One woman who likes being overweight wrote to Ann Landers as follows:

"Dear Ann Landers: I'm burning over that letter from the screwball who considers herself an authority on overweight women. That nitwit should not be suggesting psychiatric help for fat ladies, she should go to a psychiatrist herself and find out why she is so hostile.

"A person can't pick up a magazine or a newspaper anymore without being hit in the eyes with an article on why women overeat. These articles give the impression that overweight people are mentally ill or they feel rejected and unloved and food is their source of comfort and solace.

"God gave us taste buds because He wanted us to enjoy food. I am overweight because I love to cook and I can eat a meal just 'tasting'. I refuse to apologize for my size and I don't hide in the house. My husband loves me the way I am and he has never suggested that I go on a diet. I would rather be 20 pounds overweight than ruin my health with pills and end up looking like a broomstick with hair."

Why Do You Overeat?

—It is undeniably true that many people overeat as an escape from a disagreeable life situation. It is also true that they may feel unloved.

—Children sometimes overeat to satisfy a nagging or over-indulgent mother.

—Adults may overeat because of loneliness or lack of interest in life. Senior citizens, if they live alone, may not eat enough; on the other hand they may eat too much. I know an elderly woman, who upon awakening, begins deciding what she is going to eat for the day merely because she has no other interest. She *lives to eat.* An interest in others, or a new hobby, or some volunteer work would quickly cure this food-fixation.

—Some people dislike their work and overeat for con-solation.

—Others, and this is common, are stress ridden and overeat for compensation.

—Rewarding yourself with food or drink for bad luck, rejection or lack of love, appreciation, or attention from others, or other emotional disturbances is one of the easiest ways to gain weight. One woman, a successful wife and mother, really enjoyed her role. She was a former model, beautiful, with a perfect figure. She was admired by all, including her husband. Due to circumstances beyond her control, her husband left her. She lost interest in her appearance, ate constantly to forget her grief and now looks like a stuffed pin cushion. Her interest in her children also waned and had she not given in to psycho-logically negative influences, she could have had her choice of suitors. But she has lost all interest in life except eating for consolation.

Again, finding a new interest in life, perhaps helping others to replace self-pity, would solve the problem for those living in an emotional vacuum.

—There are also other simple reasons for over-eating. Some people cannot bear to see food wasted and they gobble up everything in sight whether they are hungry or not. Probably these people were always urged, as children, to clean up their plates.

—Some people consider food as a sign of prosperity. One woman I know is grossly overweight. Although she tries every diet which comes along, she doesn't stick with it long. She and her husband own a restaurant and she supervises the food daily. Her will power holds out only so long and then she can't resist the food around her. But there is a reason. This woman was rejected by her mother when she was a small girl and placed in an orphanage. She had little to eat in the institution which was run on a tight budget. So she admits that the cause of her overweight is a double problem: an old grievance of feeling unwanted by her mother, and the fact that she was often hungry simply because there was a scarcity of food. My guess is that after her marriage, she was the deciding factor in choosing a restaurant as a family business. She loves food; she loves to cook and the restaurant is a big success. She is fat, but beautiful. And perhaps it is better for her to stay that way, who knows?

What About Hypnosis?

Does hypnosis work for reducers? Sometimes, sometimes not. If a person does not wish to overcome an emotional block to success, hypnosis, which aims at reconditioning the subconscious mind, may prove useless. The woman I have just mentioned submitted to hypnosis by a successful doctor because it had helped others lose weight. She, however, did not lose one ounce!

Do Reducing Drugs Help?

What about reducing pills for people who have no will power? Wouldn't they solve the problem? If you take reducing drugs, either with your doctor's permission or without it, watch it! Reports indicate that reducing drugs, including appetite depressants, may increase the pulse rate and cause shakiness in some people. Henry Brill, M.D., states: "Over-use can result in excessive beating of the heart, high blood pressure, nervousness, emotional tension, even hallucinations."

James B. Landis, of a well-known drug company, warns that even pep pills can affect the appetite center of the brain and may cause a psychosis similar to schizophrenia.

The American Medical Association warns that diet pills, including thyroid, hormones, digitalis and diuretics, may not work and can be dangerous. At least 60 deaths have resulted from taking diet pills.

Is Overweight Inherited?

Some of you may blame your tendency to be overweight on your inheritance. It could be. Genes are a factor. Dr. Jean Mayer, of Harvard University, states that certain animals have a tendency to put on more weight than others, even though the diet is identical with animals which are not overweight. If your parents and grandparents tended toward fat, it may be a genetic inheritance; or it may be due to the fact that the love for fat-producing food runs in the family. The German diet, for example, produces more corpulence, usually, than the Scandinavian diet. And because of national inheritances, some foods agree better with some people.

The Scandinavians have thrived on sea foods for generations. The Italians, living in their warm, sunny climate, thrive on fruits and vegetables. Orientals have subsisted on refined rice for centuries with no noticeable bad effects, whereas others find it a nutritionally inadequate food. (Orientals do fortify their diet with other foods.)

Your body type is another consideration. Some types just naturally gain weight more easily than others. If you are one, your eating must, of course, differ from those who can eat anything they wish without gaining.

What About Your Frame?

Don't jump to conclusions that you are overweight because the height-weight chart says you should weigh so-and-so. The age-height-weight tables are not absolute. Some take into account the size of your frame; others do not. If you have a larger frame and heavier bones, obviously your weight, as judged by the weight of your frame and bones, will be influenced. You may be overweight, according to the chart, but not fat. A reducing diet is not for you.

How About Your Metabolism?

You have heard again and again the advice, "Consult your doctor before going on a reducing diet." There are good reasons for this. One reason is, though it usually occurs in the minority, that there are physical disturbances which can cause overweight. This is often the cause in the extremely fat person. It may be due to glandular imbalance, dysfunction of the brain center regulating food intake, or a metabolic disturbance. In the latter case, the fat person may not digest or assimilate his food properly.

I know of one couple in this metabolic category. The man has been greatly overweight until recently (a doctor spotted his problem and helped him trim down). His wife, who actually eats more than he does, remains a svelte size eight. In such physical disturbances, the doctor can help to establish the cause.

Glands, Exercise and Zig-Zag Dieting

Grant Gwinup, M.D., says, "Many fat persons console themselves with the idea that their glands are at fault. They are only kidding themselves; I believe glands rarely cause obesity. That rumor has persisted for more than 60 years, but it is usually untrue. Neither the pituitary nor the thyroid gland is guilty. About five million men and women today are taking thyroid pills unnecessarily. The pills do nothing for them except cause nervousness and weakness if the doses are large."

But there is another opinion. Dr. Mayer believes that the greatest cause of overweight is inactivity. Research proves this to be true with animals, as every farmer knows. He believes that self-indulgence or a combination of the above factors can cause overweight.

He—and others—deplore the on-again, off-again dieting, which Dr. Mayer terms "the rhythm method of girth control." It has been found to throw glandular machinery out of kilter in regulating the body machinery. The glands become so confused by the constant changes that they finally break down in their efficiency. Avoid see-saw dieting, he warns.

There is more to this gland business. But we will take it up later.

It is true that if you did not eat at all, you would lose weight sooner or later. It is also true that if you eat more food than you need, you will store that food and become overweight. It is a simple case of body mechanics. All foods are a source of energy (some more, some less), and energy is used up by the body either in movement or by producing heat. If less is eaten, any existing fat is taken out of storage. If more is eaten than is used, it is put into storage. Therefore, for a fat person to lose weight, he has two choices: he must either eat less, or exercise more, to keep his weight in balance. Once a desired weight is attained, the food intake and output must be balanced by checking scales regularly and adjusting eating or exercise accordingly. This will no doubt help you to maintain the weight you wish but it will not insure good health! And the goal of this book is to help you *feel well* and *look well* as well as *stay slim!* So now we are finally coming to the secret of accomplishing this goal.

Grant Gwinup, M.D., has apparently stumbled upon part of the secret: He says, "Practically every reducing diet—no matter how well it works at the start—is doomed to fail. The proof is apparent. The average person stays on a particular diet for a couple of weeks and then he or she is looking around for a new one. All diets fail after a few weeks. And for a good reason. All diets have a common basic fault."

Now comes the clincher: Dr. Gwinup says, "The fault of the reducing diets is that they are physiologically unsound and therefore unacceptable to your body."

I would like to put it more bluntly: the reason that

the average reducing diet does not work, does make you nervous and irritable, does play havoc with your skin and hair, as well as your nerves and makes you feel worse rather than better—as well as ravenously hungry, is that *it induces malnutrition* and actually starves you to death! No wonder you cannot stay on it for long! Malnutrition is now beginning to be considered a *disease* and reducing diets induce this disease. It is possible to feed your body *what it needs,* prevent that gnawing hunger, and at the same time make you *healthy as well as slim.*

If you don't believe it, there is proof in the next chapter. Once you understand this unique concept, you are on your way to success!

CHAPTER 2

Hidden Hunger

It is no accident that so many people are overweight and fighting the battle of the bulge. There is a completely logical explanation for it and once you recognize and understand it, you can change the situation. You can begin to bring your weight control problem under control *forever,* stop suffering from gnawing hunger, and feel and look better simultaneously. You will achieve a magic carpet to carry you through life with a feeling of well-being and better looks, all at one fell swoop. The changes you make will not be like discarding one reducing diet after another with disillusionment, but the new method will become a way of life. You can set it up and forget it while it works automatically for you.

This reminds me of another cocktail party, this time in Hollywood. Many stars were present. The women were all competing with each other, as usual, wearing the newest hair-do, the most exciting make-up, coiffure, and the most dramatic gown. The reason, of course, was to attract the admiring glances of the audience present, but especially to snare the admiration of the men. They were succeeding quite well until the door opened and a new guest arrived. Instantly there was a reverberation like an electric shock which ran through the male cheering section.

The new arrival was a well known star, but with a difference. She wore little or no make-up. Her skin had a rosy, natural glow. Her hair had not been coiffed in a set or artificial style, but was loose and free swinging, bouncy and beautiful. She had no doubt shampooed

11

and set it herself. She did not wear an elaborate gown, merely an attractive, becoming and simple dress. She had not planned to stay, but had dropped in between other appointments to pay her respects, dressed casually, not especially for the party as were the other women. But as long as that star was in the room, she had captured the attention of every man who followed her every move. The other women were digging their long nails into their palms with envy. Soon she was gone and when the door closed behind her, there was a ong, concerted sigh: relief from the women; disappointment from the men. A reporter who told me about this incident later analyzed the star, trying to pin down why she had made such an impact on everyone.

The reporter told me, "You know it was a matter of comparison. The other women looked like statues from the Wax Museum; no life, no verve. But the star was exuding health and vitality galore. She may not have been as beautiful as many women at that party, but her energy and freshness and obvious well-being gave her an electric magnetism which outshone every female present. It gave her an attraction that no man could resist."

How did she do it? She has since given many interviews to the press who have asked her the same question. Her answers are always the same. "My goal," she tells her listeners, "is good health. I try to put into my body the things which keep me in good health. I refuse to eat junk foods. I also refuse to drink alcohol. I, and many others, are learning that it ruins our skin and that we cannot appear before the camera to best advantage if we drink. I really believe that *we are what we eat,* and believe me I choose food to build me up, not tear me down."

She also added that she made a point of getting some outdoor exercise daily. She walks on the beach, plays tennis or swims daily. She concludes, "This program is simple. I eat natural foods, many raw foods in salads.

This, plus exercise and plenty of sleep, gives me all the stamina I need—plus. I do not take drugs, tranquilizers, or pep pills, either. I don't need them, due to the program I follow. For me it is not a now-and-then thing, but a *way of life.*" Her weight, incidentally, was not even mentioned because it is not a problem.

"There was not a woman in the room at that cocktail party," my reporter friend had told me, "who would not have changed places with her in an instant. Yet they could do exactly the same things she does with equal success."

Women (and men), who are fighting to stay attractive, are in the majority today. The reason they are not successful and are gradually going down hill is because our national food does not contain the elements to keep them well and vital. Their bodies, which need these elements, are crying out for help, creating in them a deep, gnawing hunger. The women, or the men with the paunches, begin trying to satisfy this "hidden hunger" with more and more food, which adds more and more pounds. Then, trying to lose the added, alarming weight, they turn to that "one more diet" which is more depleted, more devitalized, or more restricted than ever, and the hidden hunger becomes an overwhelming monster which tortures its victim finally into giving up and eating everything in sight.

You don't believe me that this is the cause of our national overweight? There is proof.

Stop and think. When you were born you were no doubt reasonably healthy (provided the diet of your mother was sufficient to build proper bones, hair, skin, organs, cells and glands. Birth defects are now known without a doubt to result from an inadequate diet of the pregnant mother). However, let's hope you are one of the lucky ones; that your mother's diet was reasonably adequate and that you were born with all the right spare parts. You also came into life with a certain amount of "fuel" to keep your body running for awhile. This supply, however, is not a guaranteed lifetime supply, but a *temporary* supply of nutrients present at birth. Sooner or later, it begins to run low and must be replenished. This is why babies start life drinking milk; it supplies much needed calcium for growing bones, and other nutrients for growth. It supplies fat and protein, too, and babies in under-privileged countries who do not have milk (or their mothers, if they nurse them, do not have the right nutrients in breast milk) become scrawny, ill, and often die only because they do not get enough nutritious "fuel" to supply the needs of their bodies.

Scientists have analyzed the human body and discovered that it is made of a minimum of 60 and a maximum of 103 elements. If *any* of these elements is missing from your body, either at the beginning of life, or afterwards, when the supply is not replaced as it runs low, trouble develops. It may not be noticed immediately, but sooner or later it happens. H. W. Holderby, M.D., tells us that these nutrients must *all* be constantly replaced. He says that 15 or 30 will not do the job; at least 60 or more are needed *daily*.

A nutritionist who wears glasses was asked by his audience why he wore glasses. Didn't he take the right nutrients to give him good eyesight? He answered, "I was too late. My mother's diet lacked the right nutrients before I was born. Many nutrients can reverse a health problem and I can prevent further eye trouble. But my die was cast in my mother's diet." Other defects, including weak heart, poor hearing and vision, as well as subnormal gland activity have resulted from such depletion during pregnancy. Fortunately, many of them can be helped, if not erased, after birth by correct nutrition.

The deficiency principle continues throughout life. The nutrients need to be constantly supplied *throughout* life, not only to control a weak link in your health (most people have at least one) but to prevent further breakdown in glands, organs, or cells. Deficiency diseases often take one form in one person, another in another. They usually strike in that special weak spot. Such diseases may include heart ailments, arthritis, insomnia, anemia, fatigue, and many others. But the underlying cause is the same: a lack of proper body reconstruction materials.

If you supply these missing elements or nutrients, can you reverse poor health? Thousands upon thousands of people who have tried it will shout an enthusiastic "YES." It is not that these nutrients will *cure* anything; when given to the body, they merely help the body to repair itself. Otherwise a person can become a nutritional cripple.

Is there proof of this principle? Yes. Radioactive tracers have been used to follow the pathway of these nutrients, once they are introduced into the body. If a liver product is supplied, it makes a bee-line to the liver to help it start its repair work. If heart or kidney or another glandular product is used, the same thing happens. So, as each part of the body is supplied with all the nutrients needed for health, these parts will begin to pick up what is needed and put it to work in the repair process. Sooner or later the various parts of the body begin to work more normally once more. This explains why countless people (I am one of them) have achieved health through nutritional substances. But, it also explains why, until these nutrients were supplied, there was a gnawing hidden hunger, and why, *when they are supplied,* the ravenous, gnawing hunger stops.

Now why is there so much "hidden hunger" causing people to overeat to try to satiate this uncontrollable appetite which results only in added pounds? Because most of our food either has had these important repair materials removed or because they were not there in the first place.

Bread, for example, is at the head of the list. Instead of being made of natural whole grains, as it was in the time of our ancestors, it has been plundered. First, the most nutritious delicate part of the flour is removed so that anything made of it will not spoil on the grocers' shelves and cause a loss of money for them. (They are not concerned about people's health.) Then, after some 15 *natural* vitamins, seven minerals, and many protein factors have been removed by processing, approximately six of these nutrients in synthetic form are substituted. But that isn't all. A bleach, agene, formerly used for thirty years to remove any tattle-tale gray (which actually shows that the flour is natural) was finally discontinued because it was found to give dogs running fits and cause mental deterioration. After agene was banned, another bleach was substituted: chlorine dioxide. Recent studies show that this bleach has stunted the growth of mice. As Beatrice Trum Hunter says in her magnificent book, *Consumer Beware!*, which is not afraid to tell the truth about the average food the average person eats, there seems to be some truth to the rhyme,

> "The whiter the bread
> The sooner you're dead."

This is no joke. Roger J. Williams, Ph. D., a biochemist at the University of Texas, fed enriched white bread to a group of 64 rats. After ninety days, two thirds of them were dead of malnutrition and the rest were severely stunted. What about people? Do they suffer the same fate? One writer states it succinctly: "A starved, underfed body cannot thrive. A body fed on an unbalanced or insufficient diet becomes ill. Sagging muscles, skin blemishes, scurvy, rheumatism, *overweight,* and many other ailments can be traced to inadequate diets. A body fed on 'garbage' becomes a soggy, pitiful thing. A diet of whole natural food is necessary to health."

So a diet of whole foods, containing all nutrients which nature grew there, is the most valuable, and it is the cheapest way in the long run to stay well. It is preferable to eating refined breads and cereals, refined sugars, refined flour products, all of which cause tissue depletion because they do not contain the repair materials and therefore are considered "empty calories". People who eat them put on weight, while unknowingly allowing their body machinery to run down.

Do the manufacturers know about this? Of course they know about it! But it is to their advantage, financially, to ignore it. Do the doctors know about it? Rarely. The doctors are not taught nutrition in medical schools. So both they and the manufacturers categorically deny that there is anything wrong with our food. But ignoring a wrong doesn't make it right. And because so many people overeat because they are always hungry, their bodies are not getting the nutrients they need or crave. In this era of "empty calories" or refined and processed foods, it may take a lot of these foods to supply these needs. A woman once told me that she craved bread and ate it, slice after slice. Her weight soared. When she began making her own bread of whole grains and other body-satisfying nutrients, one slice of bread satisfied her. Her weight dropped as "hidden hunger" disappeared.

In addition to food refining, there is another reason why your food does not satisfy your appetite or your body's needs. You may feel very virtuous by deciding that from now on you will eat more wholesome foods. Because you have heard that carrots are healthful, as well as low in calories, you may head for the nearest supermarket to lay in a carrot supply. But wait! Dr. Firman E. Bear, Department of Agricultural Chemistry, Rutgers University, used an X-ray type of machine which detects and measures the precise chemical composition of a vegetable. With the help of this machine he analyzed 204 samples of vegetables harvested at the same stage of growth from various areas of the United States. The study revealed that two carrots could look exactly alike to the naked eye, but under the merciless eye of the machine, the mineral content of one vegetable was very high whereas that of a similar vegetable was practically nil. Different soils accounted for the difference in composition. *Depleted soil yielded depleted vegetables, even though the species planted were identical.* This is what the new boom in organic foods is all about. Organic foods (if they are really organic) are grown in soil which is not impoverished and which does not produce nutritionally impoverished plants, animals or people.

A dramatic, true story illustrates this principle. In the Bluegrass country of Kentucky, a large stud farm was famous for its racing horses which had unusual stamina and speed. They were famous for out-racing other horses. Then something began to happen. Fewer horses won races. Finally the successful racing horses became almost non-existent. Racing experts shrugged their shoulders and said the strain had just "run out"; there was nothing which could be done about it.

A soil expert had another idea. Suspecting that the decline of these famous horses might be connected in some way with the long usage of the fields for pasture, due to the constant over-cropping without restoration of *all* soil nutrients, the soil was examined. Sure enough, it was found to be not only severely depleted, it was also yielding depleted food for the famous line of horses. Immediately a major program of restoring the soil *naturally,* and organically (without chemicals) was undertaken. Cattle were put on the land. Their manure, plus green cover crops grown on the soil, were plowed under before planting new forage. Meanwhile, feed was imported from areas where soil was rich. Within two years, the horses showed marked improvement. Three years after that, the stable was the third highest winner of races in the entire country! The stamina of the race horses had been restored, not by drugs, or medicine, but by natural, nourishing fodder which contained all the nutrients needed for health. The average vet who now looks at a sick or listless animal will ask, "What are you feeding it?"

Meanwhile people who are eating more and more food because their body is craving more and more nutrients, are getting fatter and fatter, because they are trying to satisfy this hidden hunger or craving. It is very similar to being an alcoholic. Dr. Roger J. Williams proved this with rats. He found that the chemical composition of the rats' food is a tremendous factor in their craving for alcohol. In other words, there is a hidden hunger both in over-drinking and over-eating, according to Dr. Williams' findings.

In a wonderful little book he has written on how to control alcoholism through the nutritional approach*, Dr. Williams says, "In scores of cases we have been able to show that a rat's urge to drink is abolished by giving it a missing food element . . . Rats may stop drinking overnight when the ration is fortified with needed extra vitamins . . . If the tissues of animals or people lack any single thing, they are malnourished."

Dr. Williams has also applied this knowledge to people who, like the laboratory rats, overcame their craving for alcohol when missing nutrients were supplied. One man, a married graduate student, was plagued by a craving for alcohol to the point that he nearly gave up his studies. When Dr. Williams recommended a vitamin-mineral supplement containing the usual nutrients missing from our foods, the man lost his craving for alcohol, recovered and graduated with flying colors.

In the case of overweight, which is so similar, many reducing diets, or fad diets, merely compound the problem.

Fad Diets

Fad diets are nutritionally inadequate. They may consist of one or more foods, such as a banana diet, a rice diet, etc. One physician and one dentist told me that many physical and dental illnesses in their patients began with fad diets. To be healthy, the body needs

---

*Roger J. Williams: *Alcoholism, the Nutritional Approach.* University of Texas, Austin, Texas, 1959.

at least 60 nutrients *every day*. A single food does *not* contain them all. Prisoners of war, restricted to one or more foods, developed deficiencies from which they never recovered. Dr. Robert McCarrison, the late internationally respected nutritionist, found during his lifetime study of nutritional effects on animals, that all organs suffer when they are deprived of proper nutrition.

Another physician told me, "I wish you could see the results of fad diets in my patients. They *always* take a toll. It may not happen immediately, but eventually the glands, organs or cells which were starved or denied the repair materials necessary, eventually begin to break down. Usually few people turn to a completely fortified diet to compensate for the loss during a restricted, fad diet. But this is the main way in which I rescue these people and put them on the road to health again."

So to avoid that nagging hunger which either drives you almost crazy, or to drink, or to overeating and thus to overweight, it is merely a matter of avoiding the wrong foods and choosing the right ones your body is crying for.

Which Reducing Diet Is Best?

Dr. Jean Mayer says, "A 'good' reducing diet is one in which the patient does not become too hungry." I add that a good reducing diet should also be a way of life, not a state of panic. It should provide all the nutrients the body needs for health, be simple and satisfying for *you* so that once you have planned and adopted it, you can turn your attention to other things. It should not be a goal in itself, but a means to a better life.

Many people who starve themselves to get thin develop a water retention problem, since the body is apparently trying to compensate with water stored for the loss of food. A friend of mine was fighting overweight, a water retention problem, *and* a craving for wine. When she added the nutrients which were missing from her diet, the water retention disappeared; so did the craving for wine—she could take it or leave it—and her weight remained constant. She is now one person who can get into the same dress she wore 20 years ago. In addition, she has abundant energy, is beautiful, and though a grandmother, looks younger than her daughter.

Now let's see how to choose health-building, weight-losing foods.

CHAPTER 3

Calories or Carbohydrates?

Calories are out! Carbohydrates are in! This means that calorie counting, which is as old as the hills, is now out of date because it is not the complete answer. Some people insist that they eat "like a bird" and are still fat. This is undoubtedly true for many people who, although they are on a starvation diet, calorie-wise, continue to retain their over-weight or even gain more.

It is true that some people can stay on a daily 1200 calorie diet and they will lose about two pounds a week. However, there are others who merely suffer from a bigger appetite, weakness, and no change in dimensions at all. Because calorie counting is unpleasant to follow and can cause hunger, it is now giving way to carbohydrate counting. On a carbohydrate counting diet, one need not suffer from hunger at all because it is possible to eat satisfying, as well as health building meals, while losing weight. Carlton Fredericks, Ph.D., says, "On this diet, if you follow it *exactly,* you would lose from seven to 14 pounds a month."

The Low-Calorie Diet

Bernard A. Bellew, M.D., states that calorie counting is inaccurate and fallible. Dr. Richard Mackarness says, "It does not work for the majority of over-weights." The March, 1971, issue of *The American Journal of Clinical Nutrition* agrees.

The Low Carbohydrate Diet

The low carbohydrate diet has been known by many names: "The Drinking Man's Diet," "The Calories Don't Count Diet," "The Stefansson Diet," "The DuPont Diet," and the most recent, "The Air Force Diet." The U.S. Air Force Academy Diet says, "This is a diet designed for those people who have difficulty losing weight on the usual low-calorie diet. It works by restricting carbohydrate intake, thereby causing the body to burn fat for energy, instead."

In order to follow the low carbohydrate diet, you do not have to do any arithmetic as you do in calorie counting. It is all done for you in a chart which lists the number of grams per carbohydrate. You must just be sure that your daily intake of carbohydrates does not exceed 60 grams.

You will find a complete carbohydrate gram counter at the end of this book. You will notice that in some instances, calories and carbohydrates are alike; such foods as pies, cakes, and rich desserts are high in both calories and carbohydrates. But on a low carbohydrate diet you will find that you may eat all the meat, fat, cheese, eggs, and moderate amounts of most vegetables you wish. This means you can eat satisfying meals, without hunger and still lose weight.

Most carbohydrate counters are the same. All state: "To be successful you must restrict your carbohydrate intake to 60 grams or less a day." However, some carbohydrates, like calories, are "empty" of nutrients. The carbohydrate counter in this book is different from all others in that it stresses carbohydrates (they are coded) which are health building. So when you choose your 60 grams—or less—from the list, you are choosing health building instead of devitalizing foods! In other words, you will only put into your body foods which build you up, not tear you down. Fortunately, most health building foods which furnish necessary nutrients are not the weight makers. It is thus possible to get rid of excess fat without depleting your tissues or draining your precious energy or vitality.

Now, which are the carbohydrates? They are the mischief makers. They include sugar in all forms (candy, pie, cake, puddings, jams, syrups, jellies, and most alcoholic drinks except dry wine). These carbohydrates can cause all manner of trouble besides overweight. Sugar and sugar products have been found to cause tooth decay, nervousness (they use up B vitamins which help support the nerves), heart trouble, diabetes, and the "new" disease from which almost everyone suffers, hypoglycemia, better known as low blood sugar.

You may ask, if sugar is so bad for you, why not use the artificial sweeteners as well as saccharin? Recent findings reveal that the artificial sweeteners can have even worse effects. One doctor believes they are far worse than sugar. And why, if one has low blood sugar, shouldn't you eat more sugar to raise the sugar level? This is a myth, similar to the one that sugar gives you energy. *All food supplies energy.* But it is what certain food does to you *after* you eat it that is important. Carbohydrates, including sugary foods, do give you quick energy, but it is not lasting energy.

At first you have an undeniably quick pick-up of energy which makes you feel wonderful. Even doctors mistakenly recommend a candy bar when you suffer from frequent fatigue. Unfortunately, this only makes things worse. After you have eaten a sugar food, and experienced the temporary lift, because it has raised your blood sugar temporarily, suddenly that sugar level nose dives and you feel worse than ever. Now you have a craving for more sugar and you soon become a "sugar-holic." Later you may develop all manner of peculiar symptoms such as irritability, shakiness, weakness, light-headedness, even blackouts. Nutritionists and nutritional doctors consider sugar and sugar foods a menace. Many cases of hypoglycemia are going undiagnosed because few doctors understand the disease. But believe me, the people are finding out. There are now "Hypoglycemics Anonymous" springing up. Some people have even been committed to an institution when all that was wrong with them was hypoglycemia (the opposite of diabetes). It was often caused by too many carbohydrates, usually sugar in some form.

There are other types of carbohydrates. These include starchy foods made of white flour, such as white bread, spaghetti, white rice; and alcoholic drinks, excepting dry wine. (We will talk about wine drinking in a minute.) *All Carbohydrates Are Habit Forming!* Whether it is sugar, bread, or alcohol, the more you have, the more you want. The converse is true: the less you have, the less you want. It is as easy as that. Everybody knows that one drink leads to another, but few people know that one candy bar or one dessert creates a craving for more.

I have told in my book, *Stay Young Longer,* of a friend who discovered this truth when her son became a diabetic. The entire family gave up sweets in order not to make the boy feel left out when desserts were served. The family soon substituted fresh fruits and actually began to feel better. (Beware of dried fruits. They are better than none, but they are full of concentrated sugar, even though in natural form.) At any rate, the wife, like the rest of the family, began to lose her sweet tooth. Eating less sugar, she craved less, thus ate less.

Sometime later she visited her mother in the midwest, in the home where she had grown up. Her mother out-did herself by making all the favorites the girl had once enjoyed: pies, and cakes, and puddings. In each case the young woman took one bite, and pushed it away. She could eat no more. Her mother was astounded as well as crestfallen. "What is the matter with that dessert?" she asked.

Her daughter answered, "It is just too sweet, mother, I cannot eat it!"

"But," her mother said, "it is exactly the same recipe I have always used." This was true, but the daughter had overcome her craving and taste for sugar, and no longer required as much.

So to lose your sweet tooth, don't try to perpetuate it by taking artificial sweeteners. Cut sweetening down, little by little, until you do not need sugar. You will get so you don't even miss it, except once in a long while, and it has happened to everyone who has begun the new way of eating. You may see someone eating an ice cream sundae, or a luscious looking piece of cake. You are suddenly reminded of the good old days and are seized with an overwhelming desire to splurge.

O.K., go ahead and splurge. It won't kill you, but you are in for a big surprise. To begin with, it won't taste as you thought it was going to. And after you eat it, if you do, you will begin feeling distinctly uncomfortable—full and almost nauseous. The young woman mentioned above told me that this happened to her. Once, at a party, she accepted a delicious looking piece of apple pie. She took one bite, and then another, only to be polite, not because she really wanted it. She told me, "Suddenly, I was in trouble. I couldn't digest that pie; I felt like upchucking it. I learned my lesson. After that, if a hostess offered me a rich dessert, I merely said no, that I no longer eat desserts."

Hostesses are no longer offended if you say this. Everyone seems to be on some kind of a diet these days, so no one is surprised. If I am eating in a restaurant and the waitress asks me if I want to try that delicious lemon chiffon pie, I say, "No, thank you. Don't tempt me. I am watching my waistline." She usually smiles and says she understands, and that is that.

But sugars and desserts, and alcoholic drinks are not the only habit-forming foods. There is bread! This does not necessarily mean a loaf, or a slice of bread. It can mean hot rolls, biscuits, sandwiches, doughnuts, sweet rolls, a "Danish," or coffee cake, hot cakes, waffles, and the like. These are starches, still a form of carbohydrates. And are they habit forming!

If you must eat a piece of bread, be sure it is whole grain. And if so, many people can handle it with no problem. Like the woman I mentioned earlier, one slice of this type of bread satisfied her, whereas the hidden hunger created by the empty calorie (or empty carbohydrate) bread did not. But there are those who cannot handle bread at all. Ruth Pfahler, an expert on reducing diets, has this to say about starchy, carbohydrate foods such as bread, "In eighteen years experience of reducing hundreds and hundreds of people, I have found one common denominator. People with excess weight from the waist down (big hips and thighs) eat too many sweets. People with excess weight in the abdomen consume too many starchy foods.

"If you want to lose particularly through the abdomen, you must cut out bread in all forms! It is not the calories, it is what bread does to your stomach. If you need convincing, put a piece of bread in a pie pan, pour water over it and later go back to that bread! It has swollen three times its size, and that is exactly what it does to your stomach. It causes fat stomachs and thick waistlines."

Well, much as I hate to admit it, I am one of these people. If I eat one piece of bread, I soon develop a spare tire around the middle. While I am eating bread, I crave it. Once I break the habit, I lose the craving. It is hard at first, just as it is to cut down, or out, man-made sweets (fresh fruit is O.K.). But it *can* be done easily by doing it gradually, using a little less each day.

Are potatoes as bad? NO! Potatoes have been maligned. They are a starch food, yes, but not a man-made starch. They contain protein and vitamin C, providing they have not been converted into instant potatoes before you eat them. Sometimes it is the gravy that gives the poor potato its unearned bad name. There is nothing better than a fresh, hot baked potato, with a dollop of butter on it. (Butter is permitted on a low carbohydrate diet.) This is why you will find it rated high on the gram counter. Choose potato over a piece of white bread, and you have a health food to help make up your 60 grams.

Now for that wine. You will find on the counter that dry wines are a mere 1 gram per 3½ oz. glass. This is heaven to the drinker! It does not mean that you can go overboard and drink the whole bottle; it is just as easy to become a wino as an alcoholic. But there is actually a medical study which reported that people who drank this much (and no more) wine with their evening meal, lost weight! The explanation is not clear. The acid may help the digestion so that less food is required. Red wine has more iron than white wine, but either is acceptable if dry. And sometimes elderly people who have little to look forward to find a glass of dry wine a real treat at the end of the day. This can take the place of a cocktail. If you want to stretch the 3½ oz., pour it over the rocks.

Now back to the low carbohydrate diet and its values. Protein, in any form, or some fat, will keep hunger at bay and energy up, whereas carbohydrates cause hunger plus a severe fluctuation of energy. A recent Japanese study tried a reducing diet which was high in protein, moderate in fat, and low in carbohydrate on overweight people. The diet also included *all nutrients* and as little sugar as possible. All subjects who followed this diet lost weight and remained healthy.

One warning: although the directions with the low carbohydrate diet state that one should take 60 grams or less, don't go overboard and think you will get thin faster if you give up all carbohydrates. You may find yourself lying flat on your face, or feeling other peculiar symptoms. The body needs some carbohydrates, perhaps to help the digestion of other factors. So though you may go a little below the 60 grams allowed you, don't try to beat the system. You will only upset your body and wish you hadn't.

The carbohydrate counter is ready to go. You may start on it today before you have finished reading this book. To build up your health, as you are losing weight, be sure to use the recommended carbohydrates, rather than the man-made ones, which are "empty" of nutrients. Keep a daily score card and tally the grams as you go. Person after person has found success with this type of weight control. It has definitely worked for me, too.

To summarize, the one diet which seems to be successful for more people than any other is comparatively new: the low carbohydrate diet. It deserves your full attention and is definitely worth a fair and prolonged trial. It not only helps most people reduce, but helps them stay healthy. Carbohydrates are mainly starches and sweets. Excess carbohydrates are stored as fat in the body (and flabby fat at that). Protein, on the other hand, feeds muscles and makes them firm. Carbohydrates have also been implicated in tooth decay, heart disease, fatigue and hypoglycemia.

The theory of the low carbohydrate diet is that by eating 60 grams or less of carbohydrates per day, fat in the body is burned up, not stored. There is no limit to many types of calories (you will find some nice surprises, believe me) and the diet restricts carbohydrates only. It is easy, fun, and rewarding. Scientific studies galore confirm its success.

Bernard A. Bellew, M.D., a staunch believer in the low carbohydrate diet, says you can even go on an eating binge now and then on this diet and still stay slim. So give it a try! Any diet should be coupled with nutritional supplements for health insurance, and the low carbohydrate diet is no exception.

In the next chapter we will take a look at vitamins.

Chapter 4

Should You Take Vitamins?

In this day and age, when food is so highly processed and so many natural elements are removed, it is my opinion, as well as that of nutritionists and nutritional doctors, that everyone needs vitamins, providing they are the right kind and taken in the right way.

To begin with, *natural* vitamins are not chemicals, but merely condensed food. For reducers, it saves eating many pounds of food. Someone asked Barbara Cartland, a nutrition columnist in England, "Is there danger of taking too many vitamins?"

Miss Cartland answered, "No! You can't take too many natural vitamins, which are food, not medicine. They are what should be on your plate, but owing to modern conditions: chemicals in the soil, the air, and the water, as well as vitamins being destroyed by processing, refrigerating and bad cooking, they are missing.

"You must supplement your diet. You eat every day, you therefore take your vitamins every day. It's not really a lot. Put all you eat in one day in a bucket, then put the vitamins you need in a small saucer. You will then see how few you have taken in proportion to all you consume."

Why don't more doctors advise you to take vitamins? The answer is the same I gave you before. Doctors are not taught nutrition in medical school and it is actually true that many patients, who are interested in and reading about vitamins in order to learn their values, know more about them than many doctors.

The need for vitamins today did not exist in the time

of our ancestors. To begin with, our ancestors raised their own organic food with all the nutrients present and at that time there were no TV dinners, instant mixes, enriched bread or cereals. All food was *natural* and *whole*. Not so today. Our food has been tampered with so that our ancestors would never recognize it. It is torn apart, overheated, kept too long in cold storage, and subjected to removal of many of the most important nutrients.

It is then subjected to all sorts of camouflage: artificial coloring, artificial flavorings, preservatives, softeners, emulsifiers, alkalizers, acidifiers, hormones, dyes, antioxidants, hydrogenators (as in hydrogenated fats). All told there are some 3,000 additives allowed in our foods! Tests with animals show many of them are not safe, but the government refuses to ban them, sometimes for political, sometimes for financial reasons. Again, this may be why overweight is such a common problem. People are filling their stomachs with this junk, which is bulk only, instead of real, nourishing, wholesome food. If you don't believe it, read your labels on everything you buy. If it carries the name of a chemical you cannot pronounce, don't buy the product! No wonder we have hidden hunger, over-eat and need vitamins to supply the missing nutrients.

But there is still another reason why most people need vitamins these days. We are living in an era of stress; wars, the threat of the bomb, rising prices and taxes, crime, riots, hi-jackers—you name it, we have it. We worry, we hurry, we live constantly surrounded by stress of all kinds.

Roger J. Williams, Ph. D., previously mentioned, found in animal studies at the University of Texas, that stresses and annoyances can increase our need to over-eat, over-drink, and also for added nutrients. The major protection necessary for our bodies is to supply these nutrients, *known and unknown,* to help maintain energy and prevent breakdown.

Many people pride themselves on the fact that they

take one vitamin here, another one there. They may have occasional, or even regular injections of vitamin B[12] and believe that they are doing all that is necessary. Well, they are only kidding themselves. Dr. Williams emphasizes that our bodies need, not single food elements, by themselves, but a complete assortment of them all! He says when he says *all*, he means *all*: that tests prove that if our diet lacks even one element, our bodies are not getting what they need. Vitamins (and minerals) work as a team. Nature grows them as a team. We should take them as a team. Otherwise, a one-sided diet will eventually exact its penalty from our body, struggling for health.

Only natural food contains all natural, known and unknown, vitamins and minerals. Synthetics do not contain them all. Synthetics have their place in temporary treatment for a disease state, but nutritional doctors feel that taken in high amounts too long, they can become the equivalent of whipping a tired horse. Natural vitamins are nothing more than concentrated food. If you must make a choice, choose whole food first, the supplements second. In food, variety is imperative. In order to get everything you need, one doctor has advised people to eat a different menu each day of the month. Too many people get into a rut and eat the same things every day. Buy yourself some paperback health-gourmet cookbooks at the health store and stretch your eating horizons. It's fun.

Which Vitamins Do What?

There are entire books written in an easy-to-understand manner, which are fascinating to read and tell what various vitamins have done for others. You will find these books listed under Suggested Reading at the end of the book. In general, here is a quickie outline:

Vitamin A: helps your skin, hair, vision and energy.

Vitamin D: is the sunshine vitamin and gives you

strong bones and teeth and the well-being you feel after being outdoors.

Vitamins B: (There are many in this family.) In general, the B vitamins calm your nerves, help your digestion, and help you sleep, feel and look better. They also help thinning hair and a host of other ailments, including mental illness.

Vitamin E: is sold as the sex vitamin in Europe. It helps circulation, helps prevent heart attacks, cold feet, hot flushes during menopause and can prevent miscarriages.

Vitamin C: prevents infections and is now being considered in Europe as a rejuvenation vitamin.

Vitamin K: helps blood to clot and prevents hemorrhaging.

Are Any of These Vitamins Considered Dangerous?

In some cases, vitamins A and D in too-high doses have been found disturbing to *some* people. The effects vary with the individual.

Take vitamin A as an example. In 1932 Mead Johnson Co. offered $15,000 as an award to anyone who could find out how much vitamin A a person needs. There were no takers, and after 13 years the offer was withdrawn. One man in England was reported by Dr. Roger J. Williams as being healthy on no vitamin A at all; and a woman in Pittsburgh, whose doctor prescribed 50,000 I.U. daily, was also apparently healthy. Many nutritionists usually settle for 25,000 international units per day, but that may or may not be the right amount for you.

Vitamin D in large doses, again for *some people,* has caused some minor disturbances. The beautiful thing is that if you should acquire any unexplained symptoms from too much A or D, all you have to do is stop taking the vitamin and the symptoms promptly subside. You have not been permanently damaged, merely temporarily inconvenienced. If you take vitamins correctly, this rarely, if ever, happens.

Synthetic vitamins in *large continued doses* can also cause trouble. This applies particularly to the B vitamins. But if you take a single B vitamin, such as B^1, B^2, B^3 (niacin), B^6, B^{12}, pantothenic acid, PABA, inositol, folic acid (all these and more are members of the vitamin B family or complex) then it is always wise to take natural foods *at the same time* which are rich in the entire B factors. I will describe these in another chapter.

How Do You Know How Many Vitamins You Need?

I am asked again and again, "What vitamins should I take, and how many?" The answer is: nobody knows. Except you. Why? There are several reasons.

Roger J. Williams, Ph.D., professor in the Department of Biochemistry, University of Texas, as well as the discoverer of the B vitamin, pantothenic acid, states that because there is such a great variety of individual difference, no single rule applies to everyone. No one has the same finger prints. But the differences do not stop here. Anatomy books show pictures of hearts and other organs of many people. None are alike in size, shape, often in location! Obviously, if these organs are different in appearance, they may also work differently. So you cannot generalize on a *physical* basis that you need the same kind and amount of nutrients as your friends, your neighbors or even the members of your family.

Besides physical differences, each person possesses different genes. If your forefathers were Scandinavian, or Italian, or Oriental, your *inherited needs* differ as previously described. So look to your ancestors and their many centuries of eating certain foods which may have conditioned your genes, thus your preference for those foods.

What about your *temperament?* Are you the emotional type or calm as a cucumber? If you are highly nervous, and/or an insomniac, it stands to reason that you are going to need more of the soothing foods such as B complex and calcium. These natural nutrients are far safer than tranquilizing drugs.

What is your *occupation,* or way of life? Is it sedentary or physically active? Do you walk to work or ride? Dr. Jean Mayer, nutritionist of Harvard University, mentioned earlier, is convinced that the amount of exercise you take determines the amount of food you should eat. Less active people, he believes, need less food, otherwise they store the excess as fat. More active people expend more physical energy and use up their fuel faster; they are rarely fat. They may need more food than their sedentary friends. Even the stress of a sedentary executive determines the amount of fuel he burns, whereas a relaxed secretary, also sedentary, may need far less than her high-strung boss. Actually, the amount of stress influences *everyone's* need for more or less nutrients.

Your size and frame is another clue. Usually a large framed, active man or woman may need more food than a smaller, less active person, but not always.

What kind of food do you eat? A farmer who is raising his own organic food, natural dairy products and other goodies, certainly doesn't need the extra vitamins needed by city people who eat refined, processed foods. Our great grandparents ate whole natural food, got plenty of exercise and had never heard of vitamins. Today, people deprived of these whole foods need vitamin supplements as insurance to fill in the gaps of the missing nutrients.

Whole foods are extremely important. They are much more complete than partial foods. Partial foods include white bread, tampered-with cereals, white sugar, white rice, instant mixes, in fact all convenience foods. Whole foods include whole grains for cereals and breads, and whole brown rice instead of white. White rice has had

B vitamins removed from its surface. Once you start using whole brown rice, which looks like and tastes like white rice, but is richer and nuttier in flavor, you will never go back to the white. It is a bit more expensive, yes, but a bargain in the long run, because you get free B vitamins, too.

One nutritional physician uses the analogy of what would happen to you if you were marooned on a desert isle. Assuming the island is in the tropics, there would be a large supply of natural (unsprayed) fruit. If you ate only the fruit itself, our doctor tells us, you would receive some minerals and a few vitamins. But if you ate the kernels as well, you would get more vitamins, more minerals. And since the skin is unsprayed, if you added the skin of soft fruits, or the underlying skin if it is a citrus fruit, he says you have a sufficiently complete diet to remain well as long as you are a castaway. You would have been subsisting on a whole food which includes, not merely a single vitamin or mineral, but a large combination of them!

So, begin your new way of life by improving your over-all eating of whole, natural foods. Wait to give it a fair trial and see how you feel. Then very slowly, begin on natural supplements. They come, grouped together, available in health stores. One capsule will not hold all you need. There is no capsule large enough! Also, there is not enough of at least one of the most expensive, but necessary vitamins: vitamin E. Otherwise, it would make the all-in-one product too expensive. So you will have to add this separately to your vitamin intake. Vitamins (and minerals) are your friends and helpers. Don't ignore them.

Also, don't deny yourself foods which rebuild your body, for fear they may make you fat. You can eat less of those which are higher in carbohydrates, but you can reserve space for them by ignoring the partial carbohydrate foods which don't do a thing for you! And don't be misled by that myth that our foods today provide

all the vitamins and minerals we need. *They Do Not!*
This is why we have to take added vitamins and minerals
and why millions are doing it because they feel better
when they do. Remember, too, that *natural* food supplements save eating tons of food, including calories and
carbohydrates!

You will have to use the trial-and-error method in
choosing the best foods and vitamin products for you.
You need not become a hypochondriac; just be intelligent
until you learn what is the best program for *you.* Watch
out for allergies. Almost everyone has at least one. Wheat
and wheat products, and chocolate are considered by
one large respected medical institution, as being the most
common. But there are others, too.

How Should You Take Your Vitamins?

Vitamins, if from natural foods, as they should be,
are food, and should be taken with food. Taking vitamins
on an empty stomach may cause discomfort because they
are so concentrated that, if taken alone, they may irritate
the stomach lining. Also, read your labels. Since not
everything can be put in one tablet or capsule, the label
may read: "The following amounts are found in *six*
tablets daily." This means, that to get everything in the
necessary amounts, you do not take one tablet or capsule
only, but six, usually dividing them throughout the day,
probably two with each meal. People who do not read
labels these days are missing a great deal of free educa-
tion. Unfortunately, in some products, the government
does not require the labels to state the ingredients. This
applies to ice cream and other food products as well
as cosmetics. This should not be. For the protection of
the consumer, everyone should know what he is using
in or on his body.

If you can find a nutritional doctor to help you, grab
him! He is rare. If you can't find one, don't despair.

Read the fascinating books listed under Suggested Reading and learn for yourself, as most of us have had to do. And remember, no one in the world has a right to dictate to you what you can and cannot eat. You know yourself and your reactions far better than anyone else who does not know you. Through self-discovery, you can work out a successful program of eating correctly, and taking the right supplements, so that you can control your weight and stay well too.

Vitamins are not the only important supplements. Minerals are even more valuable. Let's look at them next.

CHAPTER 5

Magic Minerals

Vitamins are indeed marvelous, as you have just learned. But they still are not as marvelous as minerals, a fact which may surprise you. Why? Dr. Charles Northen, M.D., one of the earliest nutritional physicians, explained the reason many years ago. He said, "It is not commonly realized that the vitamins control the body's appropriation of minerals . . . in the absence of minerals *vitamins have no function.* Lacking vitamins, the system can make use of the minerals, but lacking minerals, *the vitamins are useless."*

This means that we can get along without vitamins, perhaps, but we cannot get along without minerals. The reason for this is that the human body can manufacture some of the vitamins (the B vitamins in the intestinal tract, Vitamin D from sunshine, as examples) but the body cannot manufacture its own minerals. They must be supplied by food and water. According to Bernard Spur, Ph.D., all life, whether vegetable, animal or human depends upon minerals. When they are adequately supplied, they make a strong healthy body. When they are lacking, individually, or collectively, disease can set in.

Actually, we are *made* of minerals! A person, animal or plant is a fleshy envelope made of water, air, and minerals. For instance, our bones and teeth are largely made of calcium. The red blood cells must have sufficient iron in order to prevent anemia, etc. Did you know that many eons ago we started life as a one-celled amoeba in the ocean? Did you know that ocean water contains *all* minerals, from which the amoeba drew its nourish-

41

ment? Did you know that today your blood stream contains, by actual analysis, the identical minerals found in sea water; and that in cases of emergency doctors have given transfusions of sea water when blood for transfusions was unavailable; and the patient recovered on sea water as well as on blood transfusions?

The public, even the doctors, seemed to have forgotten this. In the 1930's vitamins were "discovered" and everyone became so excited about them they forgot all about the minerals which had long been known. So the vitamins stole the limelight from the minerals at that time and are still doing so. We may be looking frantically for health in the wrong direction. Vitamins play their part, of course, but the minerals liberate the vitamins to do their work, so they must be given *first* consideration in acquiring or maintaining health.

Dr. Fritz Kahn tells us that if a human being were squeezed like a lemon, at least 11 gallons of sea water would be obtained with the same minerals and in the same proportion as ocean water: 80% sodium, 4% calcium, 4% potassium, 2% magnesium, plus numerous trace minerals found in both the healthy human body and sea water.

B. A. Howard, in his "Formula for a Human Body" says that in the body, "there is enough water to fill a 10 gallon barrel, enough fat to make 7 bars of soap, enough carbon to make 9,000 lead pencils, enough iron to make one medium sized nail, enough calcium (lime) to whitewash a chicken coop, as well as small quantities of other major and trace minerals. Take these ingredients, combine in the right proportions, and the result apparently is a man."

If these minerals are in short supply, trouble results and health is threatened. We know that rats, guinea pigs and other animals can be diseased, or returned to health, by *controlling the minerals only in their food.* There are many amazing reported cases of health regeneration from adding minerals, alone, to the diet.

There are two kinds of minerals—major and trace. The major minerals are those which are needed in larger amounts, such as calcium, magnesium and iron. The trace minerals are those which occur in the body or in certain foods in tiny amounts or traces only, thus this is where they get their name. Iodine is an example of a trace mineral. Only a small amount of it is needed, but that small amount is absolutely necessary for energy, health of the thyroid and other functions. Those who are deficient in iodine lack vitality and gain weight easily. Unless a doctor prescribes iodine for you, it is safer to take it in balance in the several natural sources I will mention later.

What do some of the other minerals do? You already know that iron is necessary for pep, that good-to-be alive feeling. It is also necessary for pink cheeks, rosy lips, and bright eyes. People with plenty of iron may look and act more like our star who captivated the Hollywood cocktail party. Those who are deficient in iron are pale, wan and droopy. Of course, one way for women to lose iron is through their monthly periods. Again, although iron can be taken separately, it is not always easily assimilated. There are also some forms of iron which are downright dangerous. Organic iron is safer than inorganic iron. But in addition, other nutrients may be needed to help its assimilation; Vitamin E helps assimilation; vitamin C is also necessary for the absorption of iron. And hydrochloric acid is a must!*

Calcium is also one of our most important minerals. It builds bones and teeth. It calms nerves. It is often used as a help for insomnia and has been called a "lullaby pill" for this reason. Many people keep a supply of calcium lactate tablets on their bedside tables and take one or more before turning off the light. If one is wakeful in the night or just *can't* get to sleep, it is perfectly safe to take more. In fact it is an absolutely safe and non-habit

*See explanation in my book, *Secrets of Health and Beauty*.

forming substitute for dangerous sleeping pills.

What about the rumor you may have heard that calcium can pile up in the joints and cause arthritis? Calcium needs acid to dissolve it in the body. Either vitamin C or hydrochloric acid (known as HCL) helps prevent the deposits from piling up in unwanted places.

People who are deficient in calcium may be victims of leg cramps, which disappear quickly when calcium is taken. They may also be irritable, cranky, nervous and hard to live with. Calcium supplements, bone meal, milk and cheese are good food sources of calcium.

Magnesium is a comparatively new mineral, and is attracting a great deal of attention. Refined foods have little or no magnesium and most people have been found deficient in it. Drinking alcohol washes it out of the body, and the lack of magnesium causes extreme irritability, even rages, shakiness and weakness, kidney stones, muscle cramps and spasms, sensitivity to noise, confusion, depression and water retention in the body. Magnesium can be taken separately in supplement form (it is available at health stores) or in the sources I will mention later.

There is one important thing you should know about magnesium: it is an antacid and should be taken *between* meals, otherwise it will interfere with the HCL manufactured by the body, which is needed for digesting protein as well as calcium.* Magnesium, however, is indeed a magic mineral.**

Two final minerals, although there are many, many others, are sodium and potassium, which are of especial interest to reducers. Potassium is a must! A lack of it can upset the entire nervous system. But even more interesting to you who are trying to lose weight, potassium works in cooperation with sodium to balance the

---

*See discussion in *Secrets of Health and Beauty*.
**Explained in my book, *Get Well Naturally*, in the chapter on magnesium therapy.

water in the body. Sodium tends to attract and hold water; potassium helps to eliminate it. Sodium (salt) is not to be feared but respected if it is taken with potassium in a completely balanced mineral source. As you will see in a later chapter, potassium and sodium can rid the body of unwanted water safely, rather than through dangerous diuretics. Food sources of potassium are green leaves (as in salads) and blackstrap molasses.

Again, however, it is far more satisfactory, as well as safer, to take these minerals in a natural source in which they occur in the right proportions.

What is the best way to get your mineral supply? There are several good sources. One is from sea water, sea plants such as kelp, or *whole* sea salt. Charles Ahlson, the late expert on the value of sea water, wrote, "Remember, all minerals are in sea water in almost direct proportion to the mineral content of our bloodstream."

Sam Roberts, M.D., uses for himself and his patients, alfalfa because the roots penetrate as deeply as 20 or more feet and develop an excellent mineral balance. He also uses kelp for his patients and himself because sea-foods and plants feed upon and absorb the minerals from ocean water, thus these substances include every mineral the body needs.

Salt

Salt should be chosen with care. Most salt is *not* whole sea salt containing all the minerals. Instead it usually contains sodium chloride only. As you have seen, sodium can cause water retention in the body. Potassium can eliminate it from the body. In sodium chloride salt only, the potassium is missing. In *whole* sea salt, the potassium is present to help balance the sodium so as to drain off the excess water. There are, of course, other minerals, too, in whole sea salt. Some salt is labelled as sea salt, but is not *whole* sea salt. It originally came from the sea, yes, but in the processing the other minerals were leached away and only the sodium chloride remains. Labels should be required to state whether the salt is whole or merely contains the single factor: sodium chloride. There are very few whole sea salts available. The government has banned them because they are not pure white, but slightly colored because of the trace minerals. If you cannot get a whole sea salt, then there are one or two salts which are next best: those mined from land salt mines, called crude rock salt. They are nearly as high in all minerals and have been found to supply all the minerals necessary for health. Both crude rock salt and whole sea salt are available at health stores.

Seaweeds

Kelp, or other seaweeds, are one of our best sources of *all* minerals. Seaweeds are able to convert inorganic elements into organic elements by the process of photosynthesis. Pure, unadulterated kelp harvested from the sea provides a rich vegetable source of all essential minerals and trace elements, plus some vitamins and protein. For example, one small 8½ grain tablet of dried kelp (the usual size tablet) will supply you with as much iodine as is found in 70 pounds of fresh vegetables and fruits; or 56 pounds of cereals, grains and nuts; or 12 pounds of eggs; or almost 2 pounds of fish. Kelp contains 22 minerals plus added trace elements.

Jacques Ménétrier, M.D., of Switzerland, states that trace element therapy by the use of seaweeds has given good results in high blood pressure, allergies, premature aging, resistance to TB and flu. Melchior T. Dikkers, Ph.D., states that seaweeds have antibiotic qualities and help to relieve constipation and intestinal as well as respiratory irritations. They have been used for hundreds of years for diarrhea. T. J. Lyel, M.D., adds that though the action of seaweed is slow, it can help mucous membranes, gout, rheumatism, dropsy and *weight loss.* It was found by researchers of McGill University in Canada, to be an antagonist to strontium 90 in the body.

Probably the most dramatic studies of using seaweed or kelp tablets with people was done by George L. Siefert, M.D., and H. Curtis Wood, M.D., both of Philadelphia. They used Pacific Ocean Kelp (Macrocystis pyrifera) in tablet form for their patients. They found that in 400 pregnant women placed on 3 kelp tablets daily, their blood count (hemoglobin) rose from 65% to 83%. The doctors also noted the following improvements:

— better color and quality of hair
— less brittle fingernails
— less bruising due to fragile capillaries
— relief in some types of skin problems

Other good results in some cases include:

— increase in virility
— definite improvement in arthritis
— relief in cases of such eye disturbances as iritis and cataracts
— less constipation
— increased sense of well being.

Kelp tablets are available at health stores.

Sea Water

As for sea water, Charles B. Ahlson, B.S., the late agronomist for the U.S. Department of Conservation Service, reports the value of giving sea water to plants, animals and people. He reports that both bursitis and arthritis have responded to drinking sea water. George W. Crane, M.D., confirms this. He says, "It is entirely possible that water soluble trace elements may prove the greatest medical innovation in preventing such ailments that have appeared in the twentieth century."

Dr. Crane tells of the effect of sea water on his 96 year old father-in-law. The old gentleman had been bedfast and chairfast for 10 years with an arthritic hip. After taking sea water for four months, Grandpa got out of his invalid chair and began hobbling around; he also perked up mentally as well as physically. Dr. Crane said, "It seemed as if some miracle had happened. Maybe ocean water is the real 'fountain of youth' for it contains all the water soluble elements on this earth." Dr. Crane is not only an M.D. but a Ph.D., and the author of the syndicated newspaper column, "The Worry Clinic." He names 22 usual diseases common today which could be prevented by taking sea water.

Most people do not drink sea water straight. They add a little to their regular drinking water. For those who insist on drinking distilled water (a procedure considered dangerous by many eminent scientists because there are no minerals present) adding 4 teaspoons of sea water to ½ gallon of distilled water restores the missing minerals somewhat and does not interfere with the flavor. But beware of getting sea water yourself from the ocean's edge if near civilization! It can be contaminated. It should be obtained from a fisherman 30 or more miles out at sea from the greatest depth possible. It can also be bought from health stores in filtered, unheated form. Boiling or other processing removes many of its minerals.

Brewer's Yeast

Another source of minerals, plus added factors, is brewer's yeast. It contains at least 9 B vitamins (probably more), 16 amino acids (protein factors) and the minerals: calcium, phosphorus, potassium, magnesium, silicon, copper, manganese, zinc, aluminum, sodium, iron, tin, boron, gold and silver. Some of these minerals appear to be no-no's but in this form are not to be feared but welcomed. They occur in organic form and may assist the assimilation of the other minerals. Brewer's yeast is available at health stores.

New Chelated Minerals

Some minerals come in a new and exciting form known as chelated minerals (pronounced kee-lāted). Both Dr. M. L. Scott of Cornell University and Harvey Ashmead, Ph.D., Ph.G., and a veterinarian, have found that chelated minerals are three times better assimilated than ordinary inorganic minerals. Tests with hens given chelated minerals showed that the hens laid more eggs, and experiments with 200,000 animals—horses, cows, pigs and sheep—show that these new chelated minerals produce better mineral assimilation, better mineral balance, better growth of young animals and in some cases reduction of disease. John J. Miller, Ph.D., has done pioneer work with the chelates especially on humans.

What is meant by chelation? It is a complex process to describe, but simply stated, is merely blending a mineral with a protein factor so that the body can assimilate it better and faster. The chelated minerals do not contain all the minerals, both major and trace, but many of the important ones: calcium, phosphorus, magnesium, potassium, manganese, iron, zinc, copper, iodine and cobalt. Chelating them has changed them from inorganic (insoluble) to organic (soluble), hence their high rate of absorption.

Chelated minerals are of especial help in protecting against the toxicity of heavy metal poisoning, as I will explain shortly.

Many doctors are now sending samples of human hair to be analyzed to a laboratory which can determine from the hair what minerals the patient lacks. However, if you take minerals in the sources which include them all, which I am describing, you should have nothing to fear. Keeping up your intake constantly, and in balance, should insure an adequate supply.

Liquid Minerals

One means of getting *all* minerals in balance, as well as in organic form (thus easily assimilated) is from a recently discovered source of all minerals which is creating a great deal of excitement. These minerals are in liquid form and not man-made or combined, but in a naturally balanced form. They have been found in a number of mines, formerly dried up inland sea beds, in which there are layers upon layers of dried kelp, plus the remains and bones and shells of sea fossils. These dried sea deposits are ground to a fine powder and added to water. Because they are organic, they remain in solution; otherwise the minerals would sink to the bottom of the container which holds the solution. But the pay-off is what happens when people drink from two to six ounces of this liquid mineral solution daily.

It is as if their bodies had become like dried-out blotters, mineral-wise. They fairly soak up this form of minerals and results are noticeable, not in years, or months, but in days and a few weeks! There are thousands upon thousands of cases of people reporting improvement, many confirmed by their doctors. The first and most commonly noted improvements are a pick-up in energy; detoxification (without going on a special diet); then a feeling of well being; and emotional improvement. The people seem to shed depression and negative thinking and become happier and tend toward more constructive thinking. Then each seems to branch out and more gradually (though very quickly in some cases) notice definite improvement in his own weakest spot or specific ailment. Most people also sleep more soundly and notice that their nerves are calmer.

One young girl who wanted to become more trim before her boyfriend returned from Vietnam, took an ounce of this liquid mineral solution in juice, fifteen minutes before meals. She lost 5 pounds in one week. Another woman lost, by the same method, 40 pounds in six weeks. She both looked and felt well. The usual reducing diet is devoid of minerals and thus causes body deterioration. This is why it is imperative, when you are choosing your carbohydrates, to choose those 60 grams allotted to you daily, from the mineral rich foods: fruits, raw vegetables, whole foods and other natural sources. Your body needs these foods and by supplying them, you will find that you lose that "hidden hunger." But there is even a more important reason, as I will discuss in the following paragraph. This liquid mineral solution sells its takers on minerals by actual personal experience. This product is not available through health stores. It is available through doctors (many are taking it themselves) or to individuals only.

How to Avoid Contamination of Toxic Metals

We hear on all sides about lead poisoning (which has been found to cause brain damage among other ailments), mercury poisoning, and more recently, cadmium poisoning. We have held our breath and hoped they will go away. They won't. They now exist in the polluted air, the water, the soil and the food grown upon it. Dr. Ashmead recently made a trip by car from Salt Lake City to Chicago. He stopped at intervals to take samples of soil. He even took samples of snow in the high Rockies where there was little or no civilization. He found in his 1,000 samples, evidence of heavy metal pollution in every sample! The heavy, toxic metals are lead, mercury and cadmium. One symptom of such poisoning is an eczema between the fingers, with itching, small blisters, peeling and eventually rawness of the skin.

How can we protect ourselves? Dr. Henry Schroeder, M.D., of Dartmouth Medical School, supplies one answer. Processing of foods, says Dr. Schroeder, or food grown on impoverished soil, creates a loss of minerals. When the food is rich in the major and trace minerals, the heavy metals are resisted. So to prevent the invasion of the heavy toxic metals, the food and the body should be filled to capacity with all minerals! Dr. Schroeder says that the milling of wheat into refined flour removes 40% of the chromium, 86% of the manganese, 76% of the iron, 89% of the cobalt, 68% of the copper, 78% of the zinc, 48% of the molybdenum. Refined carbohydrates (white flour, white rice and white sugar) have had most of the minerals removed, but whole foods, whole grains and brown rice are more likely to contain the minerals in adequate amounts.

Dr. William Albrecht, a soil mineral expert, states that even these foods cannot and do not contain their full quota of minerals if the soil is deficient, as it usually is. Thus our need for organically raised foods is imperative in this new era of pollution. Dr. Schroeder believes that foods rich in trace minerals prevent accumulation of the toxic heavy metals and thus better protect the body which consumes them. And these minerals must be in balance! Minerals in the proper proportions assure use of sound bones and muscles, strong teeth, steady nerves, a keen mind, firm skin and healthy glands and organs.

Whole organic food is one source of minerals, particularly fruits and vegetables, *providing they are raised on rich mineralized soil.* But we dare not take the chance of using food as our *only* source of minerals. We must add minerals in higher concentrates from the sources I have mentioned earlier. Not only will these minerals charge your battery for better health, they will protect you against pollution from the heavy, toxic metals.

Our health is no better than our mineral balance. It is important that you realize the basic part minerals play in maintaining good health. Otherwise you suffer needlessly from mental upsets and physical ailments due to mineral starvation of the cells. Our soils and foods are so deficient that Senate Document No. 264 says, "No man of today can eat enough fruit or vegetables to supply his body with all the mineral salts that it needs for good health because his stomach isn't big enough—and we are running to big stomachs."

Thus we need minerals in supplement form, too, in addition to high mineral foods. So to avoid "hidden hunger" *and* a big stomach, look to your minerals!

CHAPTER 6

You Can Eat Fats and Stay Slim

Most people shy away from eating fat and/or cholesterol foods. Whenever I hear someone say smugly, "I
am on a low cholesterol diet," I feel like blowing my
top, and often do. The low cholesterol diet is a snare
and delusion and it went out of date years ago. When
I say this to people, they say, "But my doctor advised
it!" I am sorry, but doctors are so swamped these days
that they rarely have time to read, especially in the field
of nutrition. So they haven't yet caught up with the
news that a low cholesterol diet is a no-no. And here
is why.

My bewildered listeners have asked, "But isn't cholesterol dangerous?" Of course it can be dangerous, but
refusing to eat foods containing it is more dangerous.
If you don't eat cholesterol, your body still manufactures
it. It is necessary for the good performance of your sex
glands, is involved in bile salts production and the natural
assimilation of vitamin D when formed on the skin by
sunshine.

Doesn't cholesterol from food cause the blood's cholesterol to rise, leading to heart attacks? Not necessarily.
Cholesterol has been found to go up during stress periods
or worry (accountants have a higher cholesterol at income tax time; probably their clients do too). Exercise can lower cholesterol. Excessive sugar and smoking
have been found to raise it. J. D. Ratcliffe, writing in
Reader's Digest, November 1964, in his article, "Cholesterol: Guilty or Not Guilty?" states, "Many physicians
are today questioning the importance of cholesterol as

a leading factor in the heart disease problem. Although high blood levels of cholesterol are usually found in people with heart trouble, there is a growing suspicion that this may be not cause and effect, but purely associative. Says one researcher, 'We could as well note that countries which have the most telephones and flush toilets also have the most heart disease.' "

John J. Miller, Ph.D., says there may be more danger of the increased manufacture of cholesterol as a result of its being avoided in the diet, than if people ate it. Because the body has to work so hard to compensate, by making *more* cholesterol.

One of the biggest scares, and biggest myths, is that you shouldn't eat eggs for fear they will raise your cholesterol. Studies have shown that eating as many as 12 eggs a day has *not* increased the cholesterol level. As a matter of fact, eggs have a built-in cholesterol dissolver, called lecithin, which we will discuss later. Isn't cholesterol dangerous when it rises in the blood? Can it plug up the arteries so that it might lead to a coronary attack? The answer to both questions can be yes, but the way to prevent this rise is not to avoid foods which contain it. There are better and easier ways to prevent the rise of cholesterol in your body and avoid cholesterol deposits. Cholesterol is a waxy, yellowish substance which is present and needed in every cell of the body. It is especially rich in the spinal cord, nerves and brain. It makes up ten percent of the brain's weight. Even when it is completely eliminated from the diet, it still continues to circulate in the blood after it has been manufactured, mostly by your liver. It is only when it accumulates in the arteries that concern is warranted. But this concern often leads to a still more ridiculous diet: a non-fat diet.

Cholesterol is usually associated with fats, which may supply some of the raw material from which cholesterol is made. For this reason, or because many people believe that eating fat makes them fat, they go on a non-fat diet. Wrong again. This is really hazardous. Why? Let me explain.

To begin with, one study showed that a fat-free diet given to rats caused scaly feet, dandruff, sores and bleeding of the skin. Another study showed that a fat-free diet for rats produced *more,* rather than less cholesterol deposits in their arteries. A nine year study found that people who ate no fat at all had the highest blood fat levels, whereas those who ate 70% fat in their diet had the lowest. And Bucknell University found that a fat-free diet can cause gall stones. Fat is needed to make the gall bladder work. With little or no fat, it does not empty. Also, if you cut out fat, the fat soluble vitamins, A, D, E, and K cannot function in the body.

Dr. Arthur M. Master, quoted in the *Journal of the American Medical Association,* says, "Many factors other than diet play a role in coronary disease, including emotion and behavior patterns, lack of physical exercise, excessive smoking, heredity and sex. Many non-fat nutrients appear to be involved . . . In the present incomplete state of our knowledge, a drastic change in the diet is not justified."

Wilfrid E. Shute, M.D., the heart specialist, writes, "There is much evidence to suggest that there is no relationship between dietary fat and coronary artery disease . . . Similarly, the commonly held relationship between atherosclerosis (artery hardening) and coronary thrombosis has no validity."

What about that old bogey that eating fat makes you fat? Dr. Richard Mackarness, of England, says that starch and sugar (carbohydrates) are the real causes of obesity. Plenty of fat people, he says, also have low blood cholesterols and many thin people have high cholesterols. One nutritional journal reports that *there is more weight lost* on a high fat diet than on a high carbohydrate diet. The inability to utilize carbohydrates apparently converts carbohydrates to fat, whereas fat which is eaten acts as a wick to burn fat away in the body. It also staves off hunger. The high fat diet has appeared under many names. One name, the Du Pont Diet, originated because the diet was tried at the Du Pont plant under the supervision of Alfred Pennington, M.D. The results were dramatic.

Twenty men and women were allowed to eat all the meat and fat they wished. The dieters reported that they felt well, relished their meals and were never hungry between meals. Many were amazed at their increased energy; none complained of fatigue. Those who had high blood pressure at the beginning of the diet were told by their doctors that their blood pressure drop paralleled their drop in weight. These overweight men and women lost an average of 22 pounds each (some as much as 54 pounds; some as little as 9 pounds, according to their need to lose) within three and one-half months. Actually this diet was the fore-runner of the low-carbohydrate diet, since not more than 60 grams of carbohydrates, but unlimited protein, salads, butter and many fruits (including berries, orange and grapefruit, fresh pears, plums and peaches, etc.) were permitted. Oils, as in salad dressings, were encouraged.

In case you are still dubious about that old timer that eating fat makes you fat, Adelle Davis says that she had been puzzled for years by people who were not only overweight, but whose ankles, legs and thighs were swollen with water retention even though their protein intake was high. She learned that when two tablespoons of salad oil were added to their daily diet, they lost pounds. She concludes that *eating too little fat is probably a major cause of overweight.*

A friend of mine is an example. Her problem was that she stored water so that from one day to the next she could not get into the same dress; it would not fasten around her middle. If she took certain measures (we will discuss these later in the book) to get rid of the water, it receded promptly and she could wear the dress with ease. But soon, the edema returned and she was right back where she started. She tried eating more protein, fewer carbohydrates and even tried to eat "like a bird" which was practically nothing at all.

One day, when she was at her wit's end, bewailing her lot on the phone, I said, "Now, tell me everything you eat, in detail." I knew there had to be a reason. So she enumerated everything from breakfast through dinner. It included all the right things, plenty of protein and salads and fruit; few carbohydrates. Then when she wailed, "And not only do I continually store water but my skin is dry, there are cracks on my hands and even my feet, and all of the cream I rub on them does no good!," I saw a light! I remembered when I had seen her last that her skin was parchment dry, and so was her hair.

I said suddenly, "Didn't you say you eat copious green salads?" She said she did.

"What kind of dressing do you eat on them?" I asked.

She answered, "Absolutely none. If I ate French dressing or oil or even mayonnaise, I'd really get fat!"

So I told her. She was to start eating at least two tablespoons of oil daily and immediately. Within two weeks she called with enthusiasm to say she had lost two pounds, the water was staying off, and the cracks on her hands and feet were disappearing!

This brings us to oils. Which are the best ones to take?

Vegetable oils are one of our most important foods. Those higher in unsaturated fatty acids are known as poly-unsaturates (poly means more). They are safflower, corn, cod liver, sunflower, sesame and soybean oils. Since oils have a great solubilizing effect on fats, they tend to liquefy the fats in the human body. Instead of being stored as deposits which may clog the arteries, or adding extra pounds, by liquefying the fat, oils can help to remove both.

Hydrogenated fats are solid at room temperature. They can only melt at 114 degrees or higher. Unsaturated fats or oils are liquid at far below the body temperature (98.6°), usually at room temperature or about 60 degrees. Since those with a low melting point are more easily utilized by the human body, they are preferable to lard, Crisco and similar hydrogenated shortenings. According to *Prevention Magazine* (November 1958, p. 133), "Hydrogenation is a chemical process which many fats are subjected to, to solidify them. It is very destructive to valuable food elements. Margarine is a hydrogenated fat. Crisco, lard and other solid shortenings have been added to some peanut butters to keep them from separating. Practically anything you buy in the way of processed foods like crackers, bakery products, pies and pastries have been made with hydrogenated fats." This is one reason why these foods (except peanut butter) are "stop" foods on your carbohydrate counter at the end of the book. They can do you no good.

What oils are the safest? The least refined oils are the best because they contain more of the original nutrients. Oils labelled as "cold pressed" (meaning not heat treated which destroys some nutrients) are not necessarily cold pressed. But those which have been highly refined are the *least* desirable. They are highly refined in order to look pretty on the supermarket shelves or to make the flavor more bland. They are also the easiest to become rancid, once opened, because the stabilizing elements have been removed. Virgin olive oil, as well as unrefined sesame oils are probably the first choice and are usually really cold pressed. After that, the poly-unsaturates I have listed before are the most reliable if they are purchased from health stores. Safflower and corn oil are popular.

Now what about margarines? Should they be used? Are they better or worse than butter? Most margarines, in order to be firm at room temperature, contain hydrogenated oil, which is not as preferable as liquid oil. Despite their advertising, experts say that they will not lower your cholesterol. So if you use margarine, you might as well choose it mainly on the basis of taste. The better margarines are those which contain liquid oils (in addition to those hydrogenated). They must be kept under refrigeration, both at the store and at home. Also, margarines which contain no fillers or preservatives, with the exception of lecithin, are preferable.

How can you eat fats safely? Avoid hydrogenated fats. Avoid deep fat fried foods which have been cooked in oils heated and reheated many times. Potato chips are usually rancid (due to over- or reheated oil as well as exposure to air) unless they are baked. Beware of synthetic or imitation ice cream. It is often only flavored hydrogenated shortening. Ice milk is preferable. If you cannot get natural ice cream made with raw certified milk, make your own.

More precautions should include the following tips: once a bottle of oil is opened, keep it refrigerated so that it will not become rancid. After you finish your salad, drink up every last drop of oil. And when you cook with oil do not let it reach the smoking stage. Overheating oil (to the smoking point) can cause health problems.

The more oil you use, the more vitamins E and C you need, to prevent the oil's oxidation (rancidity) in the body.

Choose margarines with the least amount of hydrogenation and greatest amount of liquid oils.

And don't avoid butter! Most experts now agree that since butter is a natural product, and is completely liquid at body temperature, it should not be shunned. The fat experts I know use butter almost exclusively, with oils for cooking and for salads.

Peanut butter, if it is made of peanuts and salt only, is fine. It is a good way to use a fat as a mid-meal snack to avoid hunger as well as to prevent weight gain. Take it straight or stuff a stalk of celery with it.

But if you really wish to lower your cholesterol and prevent cholesterol plugs in your arteries, instead of going on a cholesterol-free or fat-free diet, which you know

now is not the answer, take *lecithin*. It is an excellent cholesterol emulsifier or dissolver, as well as a safe one. You can take the granules or the liquid. We will discuss both forms in the next chapter. But just to show you only one example of lecithin's value (among thousands of cases) one nutritionist conducted a study of patients with high cholesterol in which meat fat was *not* cut off, one or two eggs per day were eaten, plus butter and whole milk with heavy cream. Vegetable oil was used on salads and brewer's yeast was added to provide choline, a B vitamin. *One to three tablespoons of lecithin were taken daily. In every case, the cholesterol dropped to normal.*

So you need not fear cholesterol, now that you know how to protect yourself with lecithin. Neither should you fear eating fat, provided that the fat is eaten in moderate amounts and is the right kind of fat (not hydrogenated).

Ernest R. Reinsh, M.D., author of *Eat, Drink and Get Thin,* not only believes in the ability to reduce by the addition of fat to the diet, but he has actually reduced hundreds of patients by this method. He learned about it first hand, he says, when he was brought up on a Nebraska farm and his principal food was home-slaughtered pork—fat and rich. Instead of becoming fat on this diet, he remained trim and fit. When he was a young medic in 1923, he was called to treat a 16 year old boy in a diabetic coma. Other doctors were convinced the boy would die.

Insulin had just been discovered and at that time only about a tablespoonful of it was in existence. The patient was utilizing only half of his sugar intake and Dr. Reinsh was reading every medical journal he could find, looking for help. One medical writer believed in a high fat diet. This reminded Dr. Reinsh of his own early years on the farm, so he prescribed fat pork chops, three times daily, to his dying patient, who did *not* die! Instead, in three days, his urine was sugar free; the fatty fuel had burned away the sugar. (If you are a diabetic, don't try this on yourself without your doctor's help.)

Since then, Dr. Reinsh has used the high fat diet for successful weight loss for as many as 450 patients a month. He finds that their clothes soon become loose (although the time varies with each patient, ranging from a few weeks to 30 months, depending upon the individual and the amount of overweight). These people state that they feel well, have more energy, are not hungry and look better. In short, Dr. Reinsh believes that *"eating fat is the master key to obesity control."* It can become a lifetime diet, he says.

He gives reports of dress sizes which have decreased on the high fat diet. Here are two:

Case 1: April—Size 20½
July—Size 18½
October—Size 15
February—Size 13

Case 2: Waist size: 48″ in May; 40″ the following April

Best of all, he says, there are no sunken cheeks, hollow eyes, or shrivelled skin, or hunger. Each person feels great.

Many, many physicians and researchers now agree with Dr. Reinsh who believes that protein and fats should make up 80% of your diet; carbohydrates only 20%. He is also against carbonated drinks (even low calorie types) because he has found that they cause water retention.

This concept of fat in the diet spells the difference between the low calorie and the low carbohydrate diets. In the low calorie diet you will find fats listed as no-no's or high in calories. On the carbohydrate diet they are listed as zero, meaning you can eat all you wish. Those who have tried it have learned to their astonishment (after trying a low calorie diet without success and with gnawing hunger) that fats are not only acceptable, but the real weight losers!

CHAPTER 7

High Powered Foods

There are a few special foods which have long been called "wonder foods" or "miracle foods." This is not quite the correct terminology since it gives the impression that these foods are panaceas or will cure everything. These foods are merely richer in many nutrients than most foods. They will *not* cure everything. But they can be likened to high octane gasoline vs. regular; they deliver more punch and promote a greater output of energy. These foods have been pooh-poohed by some detractors, but the scientific analysis (which does not lie) of some of these supplies *proof* that they are richer, nutritionally, therefore can deliver more power. By incorporating these foods into your diet, you can save eating many pounds, or large amounts, of less potent foods which merely fill you up and perhaps only add unwanted weight. They are also a good value, financially, because they are full of free vitamins, minerals and amino acids (protein factors), which would cost much more were you to buy them separately.

So treat these foods with respect just as automotive specialists treat high octane gas with respect if they wish better performance from their engine. High powered foods have exactly the same effect upon your body; they deliver more punch. Now let's consider them, one by one.

Lecithin

Lecithin, as we have previously discussed, helps to

homogenize or emulsify cholesterol in the body. Lecithin is made of four factors: ordinary fat, unsaturated fatty acids, choline, (a B vitamin) and phosphorus. It is pronounced *less-i-thin* and is found in every cell of the body and should be kept there in order to help the body do its work effectively.

Because lecithin includes phosphorus, it is needed by the brain. There is an old saying, "No phosphorus, no brains." It also is a natural tranquilizer because it is found in the myelin sheath which surrounds the nerves. And it is found in the heart, bone marrow, kidneys, liver, spinal cord, blood and is extremely necessary for the male sex glands since lecithin is lost with the sperm. So lecithin should be constantly replaced to prevent a deficiency in any of these body functions. Women will be delighted to learn that it helps to distribute body weight more evenly (taking it off where you don't want it and putting it where you do) and also helps to plump up the skin. It works slowly to accomplish its wonders, but it works exceedingly well. I have reported in two of my other books, *Stay Young Longer,* and *Secrets of Health and Beauty,* of cases of heart disturbance, high cholesterol, angina, and myasthenia gravis which have responded to lecithin. *Medical World News* (May 17, 1968) also has reported that it may be helpful in preventing gallstones.

Lecithin is made from soybeans. It is available in three forms: liquid, powder and granules. The granules have been used for many years by Lester Morrison, M.D. and Adelle Davis, who recommends 3 to 6 tablespoons daily to lower a high cholesterol. She tells of a 10 year old girl with an abnormally high cholesterol level, as well as a heart condition. The girl was bedridden and had been given up by the doctors. Several tablespoons of lecithin granules were sprinkled on her salads or added to juice, and she was given vitamins B and E and unsaturated oil. She recovered; her cholesterol became normal; and she was able to return to school.

Lecithin is tasteless in any form. Hans Wohlgemuth

believes that liquid lecithin is effective in lesser amounts. He believes that 1 teaspoon taken morning and evening will be enough to overcome a deficiency and keep it in the blood at all times for protection and prevention of lecithin-deficiency disturbances. Liquid lecithin is not easy to take until you get used to it. It looks like honey, pours like honey, but there the similarity ends. It certainly does not taste like honey (it tastes like nothing). It also tends to stick to the roof of your mouth. You can try it in, or followed by a tart fruit juice. If you take it by the teaspoonful, it will stick to the spoon. I usually tip the can and estimate a teaspoonful as it flows into my mouth. Then I follow with a tart fruit juice or hot drink. (When you begin to follow the nutritional way of life, you cease to be fussy.) All types of lecithin are available at health stores.

Brewer's Yeast

Brewer's yeast is one of the biggest food finds of the century. This is not a calculated guess; it is a fact as proved with thousands upon thousands of cases of health improvement resulting from its use. It contains all of the major B vitamins (except B^{12}, which can be bred especially into it), 19 amino acids, making it a complete protein, and 18 or more minerals. Except for vitamins A, E and C, which it lacks, it can be considered a whole food. It is also an excellent reducing food.

Brewer's yeast used to be an exclusive by-product of beer. The powdered dried residue has been "killed" by heat so that it will not cause bread to rise, or by the same token feed upon your intestinal vitamins and multiply in your body, creating gas. It may cause gas for some people as any high protein food can, but the addition of hydrochloric acid (to be discussed in the next chapter) can prevent this problem. Brewer's yeast is becoming so popular as a food that it is now being made specifically for that purpose and is often called nutritional yeast. Instead of being available in powder only, it is now made in large and small flake form. Both Adelle Davis and I have listed examples galore of the improvement of health through brewer's or nutritional yeast. I will mention here only one benefit, in addition to the value of being a good reducing food. It definitely increases energy!

I have tried it myself and I have watched my children and grandchildren use it as a pick-up. My elder daughter, particularly, when she feels slightly fatigued, will automatically go to the yeast cannister, kept beside the flour, raw sugar and other staples, stir a tablespoon or so into liquid and drink it down. Within about ten minutes a pick-up is noted, which unlike the temporary lift of coffee or tea, lasts for several hours. Most people begin with a teaspoon in fruit juice or tomato juice, or hot bouillon, which blends with the slightly savory flavor of the yeast. Later, people work up gradually to ¼ cup daily and no longer bother about putting it in juice, but add it to plain water and gulp it down. As I said earlier, when you learn the benefits of these high powered foods, you are not fussy about how you take them or how they taste.

Yeast flakes are somewhat milder in flavor, but it takes more of them to provide the same equivalent of the powder. Tablets are also available but it takes 24 tablets to equal one tablespoon of yeast powder or flakes. Health stores, of course, provide all forms. Because so many people have asked me, I will state here that the variety I take is Red Star Primary yeast. My children, my grandchildren, my friends and even my pets take it and thrive on it. If you take separate B vitamins, which are almost always synthetic, it is very important to also take brewer's yeast the *same* day. The yeast is a source of *natural* B vitamins which prevents vitamin B imbalance.

Because brewer's yeast, like other protein foods, is high in phosphorus, it is advisable, when taking it, to add extra calcium. (Phosphorus, a co-worker of calcium, can take the calcium out of the body with it, leaving a calcium deficiency.) The remedy for this is easy. Combine your pound of yeast with ¼ cup of calcium lactate powder (at health or drug stores). Mix well and keep in any container. It need not be refrigerated. The calcium corrects the calcium-phosphorus imbalance so that leg or other cramps can be prevented. By having the mixture pre-mixed, it is convenient when you want to use it quickly.

Wheat Germ

Wheat germ is a superior food. The United States *Yearbook of Agriculture* (1950-51) considers it an excellent food for the following reasons: "A grain of wheat, like all seeds, contains the nutriment needed for germination and growth of the seedling. Protein, minerals, B vitamins, fat and carbohydrates are present in the right proportion . . . the germ or embryo contains a large proportion of the vitamins and protein of superior quality. White flour, as it is milled today . . . has removed the germ, also the greater part of the minerals and vitamins and much of the protein."

The 1959 U.S. *Yearbook* adds, "Losses in milling are even higher for some less familiar nutrients. For example, vitamin E is present in high concentrations in the oil of the wheat germ. Nearly all of this vitamin is removed with the germ."

This tells the entire story of wheat germ in a nutshell. And because the wheat germ is removed from bread and cereals to protect the shelf life (making them last longer on the grocer's shelves) our bread and cereals are lacking vitamin E which comes from wheat germ. Cattle, deprived of wheat germ and vitamin E have dropped dead of heart disease. Many Americans are following suit. Yet, when the wheat germ with vitamin E was restored to the cattle feed, the deaths from heart disease ceased! This valuable nutrient combination is *not* restored to the food for people. They must take it on their own. Meanwhile, the Drs. Shute, of Canada, have rehabilitated the hearts of thousands of people with vitamin E and in some cases have even got these patients to the point of mowing lawns again *without* a power mower.

Wheat germ oil has been tested by various laboratories on animals and humans especially athletes. It has been invaluable in building energy and outwitting fatigue. Both wheat germ and wheat germ oil (available from health stores) once opened, should be kept refrigerated to prevent rancidity. The raw wheat germ is less tasty but valuable for adding to baked products. The toasted type, usually vacuum packed to prevent rancidity until opened, *is* tasty and children love it when it is floated on top of milk as a cereal. It can also be used instead of bread crumbs for breading meat and vegetables, or added to meat loaf, breads, biscuits, muffins, waffles and hot cakes.

Sunflower Seeds

Seeds are excellent sources of many nutrients: vitamins, minerals and proteins. But sunflower seeds, the richest of all, take the prize. Whenever your children, or you, feel the need for a snack to hold you together until meal time, sunflower seeds are a natural. They are good for that four o'clock slump, are a perfect compliment to cocktails, and save a low blood sugar reaction if taken with coffee. They are also said to be good for the eyes and for an energy pickup.

Sunflower seeds should be eaten hulled and raw. Cooking them causes a loss of some valuable nutrients. They too, should be refrigerated upon opening because they can become rancid. If a jar or container should smell rancid, return it, explaining the reason to the health store operator. (He knows that rancid foods can be disturbing, even dangerous to health). If you are travelling and want something to nibble while you wait for a bus, train, or plane, a few sunflower seeds will give you a lift within minutes. I always carry them in my purse. For victims of hypoglycemia (low blood sugar) they are invaluable. They raise the blood sugar naturally through the protein content and are much wiser to take than something sweet.

Alfalfa

Alfalfa is one of the most complete and nutritionally rich of all foods tested. It is one of the richest foods known. In addition to a fabulously high potency of vitamins as well as minerals, it is high in protein and contains every essential amino acid. Its anti-toxin or detoxification properties surpass those of every other food tested. Although the foods tested (liver, brewer's yeast, wheat germ) also have anti-toxin properties, alfalfa's anti-toxin properties were found far superior. It has been found to provide resistance to disease and seems to help diseases which end in "itis," such as arthritis. It also helps to prevent exhaustion and provides an excellent calcium-phosphorus ratio (2:1) so that it is not necessary to add calcium to balance the phosphorus.

Alfalfa seems to be most effective when it has had the fiber removed before being pressed into tablets. It is an outstanding, natural product.

Rice Polishings

Rice polish (or rice bran) is loaded with B vitamins. It is the outer covering which has been removed from whole, brown, natural rice, the lack of which caused prisoners and chickens in a penal institution to stagger, a disturbance later diagnosed as beri-beri. When the rice polish was restored to the human and animal diet, their health returned.

Rice polish has a mild flavor and can be used as an excellent method for fortifying foods. Usually, after it is taken off the white rice, it is sold back to the public in vitamin preparations. It is less expensive, in the long run, to buy it in powder form at health stores to add it to breads, biscuits, muffins, pie crust, meat loaf, and cereals. It can be used cooked or uncooked. Cooking does not destroy its value.

Cultured Milks

The cultured milks are of great value for health. They help to stabilize the intestinal flora so that digestion is improved and many B vitamins can be synthesized in the intestines. After taking antibiotics, it is imperative to take acidophilus or one of the cultured milks, since the antibiotics kill the friendly intestinal flora which must be re-established to encourage the return of health. In Italy, doctors routinely give a cultured milk product simultaneously when prescribing antibiotics.

The cultured milks include Kefir, cultured buttermilk and yogurt. These can be purchased, but it is also possible to allow your own milk to clabber at room temperature, or with the aid of a starter, which can be purchased at health stores, and make your own. Kefir is liquid. Yogurt is more custard-like. Directions are supplied when you purchase the starter. There is some indication that powdered skim milk has been used to make yogurt more solid, but it is better to avoid using it since it is rich in galactose, an antagonist to Vitamin B^2 or riboflavin. Animals made deficient in riboflavin have developed cataracts. Yogurt may be perverted by *artificial* additives (colorings and flavorings). Countries which have used it for generations for health use it unflavored.

Blackstrap Molasses

Blackstrap molasses is another food that you hear belittled. Those who do not understand nutrition may consider blackstrap a fad. I repeat, no single food is a panacea, but blackstrap is a truly rich source of minerals and vitamins. What about other sweeteners?

White sugar contains no nutrients and is pure carbohydrate. The best form of sugar, if you must use it, is called Yellow D sugar. It is rich brown sugar made from cane molasses and contains some natural vitamins and minerals. It is called a "raw" sugar. Better than raw sugar, as a sweetening, however, is natural, unrefined, unclarified and unheated honey. If it is unprocessed and unrefined, it includes vitamins and minerals. Honey which is labelled as "pure, deluxe" and is so clear and pretty that you can read the label through it, is robbed of its nutrients. Reject it in favor of the cloudier, natural honey. That found in the comb is probably even richer, nutritionally, because it has not been tampered with in any way.

To produce molasses, a sap from the sugar cane is collected. The first extraction, after boiling, is crystallized raw sugar (see Yellow D above). Usually it is later refined into "pure" white sugar and robbed of *all* nutrients. This white sugar encourages tooth decay, low blood sugar and a host of other ailments because it *robs the body of B vitamins.*

The second extraction produces a light molasses, richer in vitamins and minerals than raw sugar. The third and last extraction, at the bottom of the barrel, so to speak, is the richest of all and is called blackstrap. Most of the nutrients have settled there. If you hear that blackstrap molasses includes straw, dirt and other extraneous material, pay no attention. This could be propaganda. It has served people well for centuries and improved health. It contains more calcium than milk, more iron than many eggs, more potassium than *any* food and is an excellent source of B vitamins. It contains no sugar at all, which is in its favor. It can be added to yogurt, used for cooking. If it is taken straight, the mouth should be rinsed immediately since *any* sticky substance encourages tooth decay. Blackstrap taken internally, has been found to recolor hair in some cases, has prevented anemia (because of its high iron content) and has even been credited with stopping falling hair.

Liver

Liver has been considered one of the best "health foods" for many years. It contains vitamin B^{12} and doctors and nutritionists advise eating it once or twice weekly. It provides protein, vitamins, minerals and energy, as proved by experiments with laboratory animals. Many doctors consider it a necessity for regaining or maintaining health. One physician says, "Adding liver to your diet invariably has resulted in a lasting improvement, often evident within a few days."

The reason that liver is so effective is that it is a depot of all vitamins and minerals taken into the body. This is a *plus* factor. But there is also a *minus* factor in our present day polluted civilization. The liver is also a filter for poisons and pesticides which can lodge there in the fatty tissues. (Pesticides are always stored in fat.) For this reason many people are afraid to eat liver these days. Fortunately, there are several solutions to the problem. Organically raised meat does not come in contact with pesticide sprays or other chemical poisons. Therefore organic liver is safer. But some people do not like liver. In this case, desiccated liver, dried at low temperature to retain the nutrients, can be taken in powder or tablet form. One company derives its liver from animals raised in Argentina, where sprays are not used. Other companies now *de-fat* their desiccated liver which removed not only the fatty tissue but the pesticides and other poisons stored there.

Liver has been given (in desiccated form) to athletes to provide stamina. It, too, has recolored some cases of prematurely gray hair. It is a powerhouse of nutrients and, in its safer forms, should be high on your list of high-power foods.

Sprouts

Many seeds and nuts are nutritionally rich. They contain vitamin E (the germ for regrowth upon planting) as well as protein, other vitamins and minerals. They are most nutritious when eaten raw, since cooking destroys much of their value. However, there is a way of using seeds which really hits the jackpot, nutritionally: Sprouts from seeds. You can sprout them at home, or buy them already sprouted at health stores, even some supermarkets. They can be germinated from any whole, unhulled seeds or beans. The most popular are mung, soy, alfalfa, and wheat. If you make them yourself, do NOT buy those seeds which are coated with fungicides, mercury or other poisons. These are usually found at seed stores. Those at the health stores are safe.

The Chinese, of course, have used bean sprouts for centuries. Sprouts can be added to salads, sandwiches, or dropped in the last minute into soups, casseroles or omelets, so that they will remain crisp and not be damaged by cooking at high heat.

Each person who sprouts seeds has his favorite method. I like mine because it is so simple and easy. Soak the seeds overnight. In the morning, drain them. Place a white paper towel in a colander. Spread the seeds, one layer thick, on the towel. Cover with another paper towel. Hold the whole thing under the water spigot and gently allow cold water to run over the towels, soaking them and the seeds. Drain again. Put the colander away in the corner of the kitchen counter and forget about it until the next morning. At this time, re-irrigate in the same way. Dampen them every morning. Within a few days the seeds will develop little "tails" or sprouts. When they are about an inch long, remove the towels, wash the sprouts and refrigerate them. If you have sprouted mung beans, or another type which has husks, merely float the sprouts, husks and all, in a full bowl of water. The husks will float to the top and you can skim them off. It is now time to start a new batch.

A friend of mine lived next door to a physician. Both had children and my friend always kept a bowl of sprouts on the table after school for the children and their friends to eat as snacks. They loved them. Later, the physician and his family moved away. After some time had passed he wrote, "As long as we lived next door to you, our children remained healthy. Since we have moved, they have been less healthy. The only way I can account for this change is that the sprouts must have contributed to their health. We are going to make them a habit in this family from now on."

There is no doubt that sprouts are nutritious because they contain a fantastic amount of vitamins B, C and E. When seeds sprout, the vitamin content increases, depending upon the vitamin, 10, 50, 100, 500 and 1,000 percent! They are one of the cheapest sources of natural (not synthetic) vitamins you can find.

Catharyn Elwood tells the full story of the increase of vitamin content of sprouts, in her book, *Feel Like a Million* (available at health stores). I am going to quote only one analysis from her book to give you an idea of how sprouting seeds increases their value.

Analysis of B Vitamins in Sprouted Oats

According to Dr. Paul Burkholder of Yale University, and reported by Catharyn Elwood in *Feel Like a Million,* the following are approximate increases in B vitamins in sprouted oats:

Niacin	500%	Folic acid	600%
Biotin	50%	Inositol	100%
Pantothenic acid	200%	Thiamin (B^1)	10%
Pyridoxine (B^6)	500%	Riboflavin (B^2)	1350%
		Nicotinic Acid (B^3)	500%

As we close this chapter on these unusual foods, don't let anyone kid you into thinking there are no such things as wonder foods. Now you know the truth.

No wonder you can eat fewer of these foods in order to get greater values. They are a gold mine for reducers!

Chapter 8

Protein—The Real Stuff of Life

The tissues of your body are composed of protein. All parts of your body are dependent upon protein in some way for survival. Lack of protein weakens your muscle tone, and makes you flabby. Without protein your facial muscles begin to droop and your skin begins to shrivel and wither. Adelle Davis says, "Since your body structure is largely protein, an under supply can bring about age with depressing speed . . . muscles lose tone, wrinkles appear, aging creeps in; and you, my dear, are going to pot."

No living being survives without protein. The word "protein" was coined by a Dutch chemist in 1839 and means "of first importance." It is the stuff of life as you will soon see, but I prefer to call it the staff of life. Bread, formerly called the staff of life, no longer qualifies. But protein does. Hear this:

— Hormones which regulate our bodies are proteins.
— Our genes are protein.
— The secretions of the thyroid gland, and the pituitary (the master gland) are proteins.
— Insulin, the secretion of the pancreas, is a protein.
— Antibodies which protect you against infection are proteins.
— Enzymes, which perform a myriad of jobs in your body, are protein.
— The red coloring matter in your blood (hemoglobin) is a protein.
— Your heart, liver, kidneys and eyes are made of protein.
— Your hair and skin are about 98% protein.

Prolonged protein deficiency can cause:

anemia	low blood sugar (hypoglycemia)
kidney disease	weakness
liver disease	wasting
peptic ulcer	high cholesterol
poor wound healing	poor circulation
lack of resistance	constipation
to infection	mental retardation in child
irritability	poor vision
fatigue	edema or water retention
low blood pressure	(reducers, please take note)
nerve instability	

In other words, you need a continuous, *daily* supply of sufficient protein in order to maintain your body at the top peak of efficiency and normalize your weight. Protein cannot be stored in the body for long. When the supply is depleted, the body is forced to feed upon itself causing tissue and muscle breakdown in all parts of it. So protein is needed every single day.

This information about protein and its effect upon the body is NEW. George K. Anderson, M.D., of the Council on Foods and Nutrition of the American Medical Association, stated in 1954 that the knowledge that protein is a preventive and curative food substance had developed only within the last few years. He stated that though there were no *noticeable* effects from a temporary deficient intake of food proteins, over a prolonged period of time, a protein deficiency could bring about the ailments I have just listed. There is no guarantee that inner changes are not taking place during a temporary deficiency. Many disturbances do not appear overnight. The damage is taking place behind scenes and can eventually erupt as a time bomb.

How much protein should one eat daily? The general recommendation is that for every 2.2 lbs. of body weight, you need 1 gram of protein (the measure of weight of proteins). If you divide your weight by 2, you will get the approximate amount of protein you need daily. (I will show you the gram equivalents for various food proteins shortly.) However, the recommended amounts of protein vary in different countries; no one can quite agree, except that pregnant women as well as those breast feeding their babies need more; people who have been ill need more (for repair purposes); and men need more than women. The recommendation in this country is 65 grams of protein daily for men, and 55 for women. Our recommendations, however, are considered low. In Sweden, hard working laborers were found to need 189 grams daily; Russian laborers, 132; German soldiers, 145; Italian laborers 115; French workmen, 135; and in England the rate for workers is 151. However, the British Medical Association believes that a realistic allowance should be between 80 and 100 grams daily for the average person.

Most people today are living on a high carbohydrate diet, which causes overweight, fatigue, irritability, and predisposition toward illness. If your diet is full of all the necessary minerals, you may need less protein. But in addition to a high carbohydrate diet (which is usually lacking in minerals) most people are also eating a low mineral diet, making sufficient protein a must for both weight control, health and vitality. You know, no doubt, that athletes are required to eat a high protein diet to provide stamina. *You* need stamina, too.

What kind of protein is best? Animal protein is similar to that of the human body, so nutritionists consider it preferable. This includes meat, fish, fowl, milk and eggs. These proteins are *complete* proteins, meaning that they contain *all* the essential protein factors, known as the amino acids. There are 22 of these amino acids; some essential, some non-essential. The body *must* have all the essential amino acids in order to synthesize protein and maintain its protein balance. Animal feeding experiments have also shown that the body needs all of the essential amino acid in *each* meal. If one or more of the essential or important amino acids is missing at that meal, it cannot be made up for by another meal even four hours later. As an example, gelatin, which you may take in water or juice is an *in*complete protein, and thus, if you take it alone, you are not getting all the amino acids your body needs at one time. If you were to combine it with bouillon (made from meat) you would have a complete protein. Soybeans as well as brewer's yeast and wheat germ are complete proteins. Most plant proteins are not complete. Here is a list of complete proteins and their equivalent in grams, showing how much you have to eat to get your daily quota of 80 grams per day, according to the British Medical Association.

Complete Proteins

	Amount	Grams of Protein
Soybean flour, low fat	1 cup	60
Wheat germ	½ cup	24
Brewer's yeast, powdered	½ cup	50
Egg	1	6
Milk, whole, skim, or buttermilk	1 qt.	32-25
Cottage cheese	½ cup	20
American or Swiss cheese	2 slices	10-12
Soybeans, cooked	½ cup	20
Meat, fish, fowl	¼ lb. (approx. 1 serving)	15-22

What about vegetarians? Can't they still be healthy without using animal protein? The answer is yes and no. Yes, if the vegetarian knows how to compute his amino acids! No, if he doesn't. Believe me, if you depend upon protein foods other than animal proteins, you have to be a brain to make the grade. The only vegetarian I have ever known who remained healthy, vital, and energetic, occasionally eats some fish and fowl and relies heavily on brewer's yeast to make up his daily protein quota. At night he takes a note-pad and pencil and figures out his number of grams as well as his amino acids for the day. If his gram count is low, he makes up the deficit before bedtime. It can be done, but it is hard work.

The best sources of vegetable proteins are legumes (certain peas and beans), seeds and sprouts, some grasses and some nuts. The soybean is the most complete protein of all vegetables. Brewer's yeast is an excellent high-protein, non-meat food. It is cheaper than meat and can be grown within days or less, whereas it takes many months to grow animals for food. The greatest drawback of vegetable protein (even brewer's yeast, unless it is especially bred to contain it) is a complete lack of vitamin B^{12}. This is serious, and vegetarians have been found to have a lower amount of B^{12} in their blood serum than non-vegetarians. A B^{12} deficiency can sneak up on you and result in pernicious anemia. Adelle Davis warns vegetarians that they are subject to pernicious anemia unless they use milk and eggs in generous amounts. She says, "People who have followed a vegetarian diet without milk or eggs for five years or longer often develop sore mouths and tongues, menstrual disturbances, and a variety of nervous symptoms including a 'needles and pins' feeling in hands and feet, neuritis, pain and stiffness in the spine and difficulty in walking."

Those who are lacto-ovo-vegetarians (meaning that they drink milk and eat eggs and other dairy products, but no meat, fish or fowl) have an excellent health record. Vegetarians who do not take these precautions often argue, "But I feel so good on beginning a vegetarian diet!" That word, "beginning" is the clue. The person is probably eating more fresh fruits and vegetables, which supply more minerals, and at first the protein shortage is not apparent. It may take months or even years for the explosion of that time bomb, but it does happen and I have seen it happen. On quick recall I can think of three people who have been vegetarians for several years. One woman is suffering from pain in the spine which continues day and night. Nothing has been found to give permanent relief. Another woman, for many years on a vegetarian diet, developed heart trouble, kidney trouble and is constantly bloated with water, making her appear overweight, which she actually isn't. She finally made her choice to discontinue vegetarianism and is feeling better and looking better. The third person, a comparatively young man, has also been on a vegetarian diet for many years. He is suffering from excruciating pains in his hands and feet, his nerves are raw, he cannot sleep but a few hours, he is in constant torment. He, too, has turned against vegetarianism, but it may be too late for repair to this nerve degeneration, a common aftermath of B^{12} deficiency. Even if these vegetarians add B^{12} at this late date, it may not be absorbed, since poor assimilation of both B^{12} and protein is a direct result of a prolonged vegetarian diet.

"But," you will say, "Our meat, fish and fowl is not fit to eat these days." You are right, not all of it. Meat is treated with hormones. Chickens are, too, and grown as quickly as possible for the market. Fish is being contaminated with mercury and pesticides which have invaded the water. The solution here is to look for organic meat and poultry (available at most health stores) and get fish which you know has come from deep sea levels. Such food is harder to get and also more expensive than the run-of-the-mill supply at supermarkets. But maintaining good health these days costs money, though not nearly as much as drugs and hospitalization. Many a family has cut its drug and other health costs by returning to good organic food. This, too, is a pitfall. Many suppliers are finding out that "organic" is a magic word and are claiming that food is organic when it is not. Health stores are the more trustworthy in this respect.

For those of you who have a distaste for meat because of your liking for animals, I will not argue except to point out that on this planet there has always been the survival of the fittest. Birds eat insects (a protein diet), big fish eat littler fish, and so on, as all nature survives.

The day may come when we will have rconditioned our genes so that animal protein will not be necessary, but for the present, I, for one, am afraid to go without it.

If you truly wish to learn how to compute amino acids and balance plant foods so that you will get a completely balanced protein intake, there is help for you. There is an excellent little book (in paperback) which tells you how to do it. It is so complicated I could not begin to summarize the method here. But you can buy the book, by Frances Moore Lappé: *Diet for a Small Planet* (published by Friends of the Earth and Ballantine Books). Study the method and by following the rules you can become a successful vegetarian, providing you also get B^{12} in some way. This is crucial. B^{12} needs an "intrinsic factor" to make its assimilation possible. This factor is now available by prescription only. There are a few brands of Vitamin B^{12} at health stores which include the B^{12} absorption factor in another form. (Read your labels.) The only other solution is to take B^{12} injections, which guarantee it reaching your blood and cells by circumventing the digestive tract where it is unlikely to be picked up. Dairy products also furnish B^{12}.

For you who are reducing, I call your attention to one other problem in following the plant combinations in order to establish a protein balance. Animal protein, or dairy products, are made almost entirely of protein. Grains, cereals, legumes (beans and peas) are higher in carbohydrates. The animal-dairy food products also contain some fat, which the body needs; the plants do not. You must make the decision whether to be firm and lean on an animal and/or dairy product diet, or risk overweight on a carbohydrate-high vegetable protein diet.

In any event, this is still not the whole story for success in order to thrive on any kind of protein. You must first digest it! Many people complain that meat (or brewer's yeast) or something else, they are not sure what, does not agree with them. They may say that either they suffer from gas or that their food just sits there in their stomach and feels like a lump, or rock or a stone. This may very possibly be due to a lack of hydrochloric acid.

HCL is a digestive acid naturally secreted in normal stomachs. It digests protein, and the minerals, calcium and iron. Without HCL you can be in trouble. Many people decide, after watching TV commercials, that they have an over-acid problem or heart burn, and take an antacid. Because the symptoms of too little acid are *exactly the same* as too much acid, it is the worst possible thing they can do. Dr. Hugh Tuckey, an expert on HCL, states that the only way to find out is to use the trial-and-error method, since few doctors understand this problem. He suggests taking an HCL tablet (he prefers HCL Betaine-plus-pepsin, from health stores) after a protein meal. If you find that lump feeling or the gas subsiding, you have solved your problem: a lack of HCL. If, on the other hand, you feel a burning sensation in your stomach, it may really be too much acid, a very rare occurrence, Dr. Tuckey says. If this happens, you simply drink a glass of water, which flushes away the extra HCL and the sensation should stop promptly.

I wish I could tell you how many people who had been uncomfortable and embarrassed by gas have written me, "Why didn't someone tell me about hydrochloric acid before? It has changed my life!"

What causes a lack of this natural digestant? Stress, anger, bickering at the table, worry before eating, as well as hustle and bustle of our daily life. It used to be that only older people, as they became older, suffered from lack of hydrochloric acid (and didn't know what to do about it). Now, stress of any kind, as well as a lack of B vitamins or protein, can be a cause at any age. Even some babies lack HCL. When a few drops of the liquid form are added to their formulas, formerly puny infants begin to thrive.

More and more people are becoming aware of the great value of HCL in helping them to digest protein *of any kind,* animal or vegetable or dairy. One nutritionally-oriented physician, who prescribes it routinely for most of his patients and witnesses the good effects, takes it himself, as I do, too. He says, "If I were marooned on a desert island and had only one nutrient to choose, I would take HCL."

If you need it and begin to use it, you will feel the same way.

CHAPTER 9

Fasting—Is It Safe?

There are many kinds of fasts. Unfortunately, people tend to lump them all together under one name. When one person speaks of a fast, he may be thinking of one kind, whereas another may be thinking of another form of fasting. There are juice fasts, fruit fasts, raw vegetable fasts, lenten fasts and water fasts. Fasts should be *labelled* so that it will be clear which type is under discussion. *All long fasts should be supervised by a doctor.*

Any fast should be chosen with care because there *are* side effects, both major and minor. An example of a minor reaction, common to any fast, was clearly evident when I was editing a magazine article written by a talented writer. Normally the author's articles were clear and convincing and I rarely had to make more than one or two corrections in the entire article. This particular article, however, dealt with the subject of fasting, and the author admitted that while he was writing it he had been on an orange juice fast for several days. He assured his readers that he felt fine, just fine. But his writing belied his assurance. It revealed fuzzy, disjointed, clouded thinking. I was forced to make a correction on nearly every line. This is because fasting detoxifies or throws off body poisons. Weakness sets in. The faster is not quite himself. One who is fasting should choose a time when he does not need to appear at his best. He will probably be weak and shaky, feel draggy and inert. Fasts have been known to make people seriously ill, even kill them. The water fast, during which one eats or drinks nothing but water, is the most dangerous of all. Actually, water fasting, also known as total fasting, can be suicidal. Why?

Those who argue that fasting dates back to biblical days, and can remove all of the poisons from the body, producing miraculous cures, forget that we are not living in biblical times. Today we are living in a totally different environment of polluted air, water and food. DDT, for example, which we have picked up along the way, has become stored in our fatty tissues (remember, all pesticides have an affinity for, and are deposited in fat). During total or water fasting, the body has nothing to eat, yet must have fuel from some source. So it turns cannibal and *feeds upon itself.* During total fasting these poisons are released suddenly into the blood stream as the fat breaks down and we poison ourselves. There are actual cases on record of people who have become seriously ill or have died on a total (water) fast.

There is another serious hazard from total fasting. Not only do our bodies contain insecticides (now a world wide problem) but strontium, another international menace, resulting from nuclear testing. During fasting, the strontium burrows deeper into the body and has no place to go except to areas with which it has the greatest affinity—the bones. People who complain of bone-tiredness, may be suffering from strontium contamination. (Kelp and calcium have been found to be antagonists to strontium, and supply a little, but not total, relief.)

Meanwhile, there are various writers and therapists who still maintain that fasting is *THE* way to health. Not in these days, it isn't. Due to heavy metal poisoning (lead, mercury, cadmium), those who urge you to fast to get poisons *out* of your body (which take nutrients away too) are merely encouraging you to invite more dangerous poisons *into* your body!

Four physicians at the University of California Department of Medicine and School of Public Health in Los Angeles, studied 11 obese patients who maintained a prolonged fast on water and vitamin pills. Serious complications developed in *every one of them.* Temporary anemia, low blood sugar (hypoglycemia) and gout were a few of the ailments noted. The problems usually disappeared after the patients began to eat again. The conclusion of the study was that prolonged water fasting is definitely hazardous.

Another report from a scientific publication told of two wrestlers who collapsed before they could take part in a wrestling match because they had been placed on a starvation diet in order to lose weight.

One dentist told me that he had observed signs of damage in the mouth (which also reflects damage in the body where we can't see it) after only three days of total fasting. I asked a nutritionally-oriented physician for his opinion on fasting. He said, "I wish you could see the deterioration in some of the body organs of my patients after total fasting."

Dr. Jean Mayer, of Harvard University, states that fasting will, indeed, cause a weight loss, but the loss will be of *protein* (which keeps you firm) instead of *fat*. This loss causes the muscles to become flabby.

It is absolutely true that we can be filled with junk from drugs, food adulterated with additives, colorings, etc., as well as undigested food (as a result of insufficient hydrochloric acid). The intestines can become clogged like a sewer and make you feel under par. It is a good idea now and then to give the body a rest and become detoxified. A modified fast would be safer than total fasting for cleansing purposes. It could be a juice, fruit or raw vegetable fast. Some people reserve one day a week and drink juices only. Other substitute fresh fruits, or fresh raw salads (unsprayed, of course), which act as housecleaners for the body. If you prolong this modified fast, be sure to take all your usual vitamins and minerals, too, since the body needs *all* nutrients *every* day. After one day of a modified fast, you may be encouraged to add more raw food to your diet. One consumer magazine said, "Generous additions of more raw fruits and vegetables to the daily diet for a period of one week to one month will usually put new spring in the step, clear the mind, improve the memory, and sensitize the taste buds . . . You feel as if you are walking on cloud seven."

Many people warn that if you have been fasting, even on a modified or detoxification fast, it is important to end your fast with care. Otherwise, the stomach, which has had a rest, may not be prepared to suddenly accommodate a heavy load. It may rebel and cause gastric disturbances. Make your transition back to a normal diet very gradual. Take a day, perhaps for fruit, then another day for fresh raw salads (chewed thoroughly) before returning to a regular diet.

Fad Diets

Fad diets can also be disastrous. This is another place where a doctor's supervision is required. A fad diet is one which may contain only one or more foods. If this is done under the watchful eye of a doctor who also supplements such a restricted diet with all the necessary nutrients in supplement form, it can serve a purpose. But it is not a safe do-it-yourself program.

One young housewife told me that she had gone on a rice (only) diet for several weeks to "purify herself." She did not add any supplements to compensate for the loss of those nutrients not supplied by rice, vitamin C in particular. This young woman became seriously ill and nearly died. Another person had similar results after a prolonged rice diet and had to be hospitalized. The patient was found to be dangerously low in vitamin C (a protection against some toxins and infections). When vitamin C was administered, together with other necessary supplements, the patient recovered. Others have not. Eating whole brown rice for no longer than three days and taking your complete array of supplements simultaneously can have various good results, perhaps as well as be a means of losing a little weight. Beyond that time, the body is forced to feed on itself, as in a total fast, in order to try to satisfy all of its many needs: proteins, minerals as well as vitamins. Beware of going on a prolonged diet of brown rice or any single food *alone.*

The highly touted grapefruit diet, said to be the Mayo Diet (the Mayo Clinic refuses to acknowledge it even as a step-child) is not necessarily a restricted diet. It does not mean that you eat grapefruit, only, but start each meal with one-half grapefruit or a glass of grapefruit juice. The rest of the diet is basically a high protein diet, except for the grapefruit, which is high in carbohydrates. In reasonable amounts grapefruit is a healthful food for some people *but not for others.* For arthritics, citrus fruits can be dynamite and increase pain.

The grapefruit diet works for some, not for others. I have known those who lost weight on it: I have known others who lost nary an ounce.

You do lose weight on fasting, partial fasting or on fad diets. But your body becomes so starved with hidden hunger for the nutrients it needs, that you are usually ravenous and soon gain back all the weight you lost.

Which Reducing Diet Is Best?

Dr. Jean Mayer says, "A good reducing diet is one in which the patient does not become too hungry."

I add that a good reducing diet should also build up the health of the dieter by providing all the nutrients the body needs. It should be simple and satisfying for *you.* The low carbohydrate diet, if you choose the right carbohydrates allowed, as well as other foods which are health building, seems to fulfill more of the requirements than any other reducing diet. More people report success with it.

Once you have planned and adopted a completely balanced reducing diet, as I have said previously, it should become not a now-and-then thing, but a *way of life.* Set it up and then turn your attention to other things. Weight control should not become an obsession, but the means to better health, better looks and a better life. Once you have achieved the desired weight, try not to let it accumulate again. It's easier to keep it off than take it off!

CHAPTER 10

Tips on Successful Reducing

Now, after hearing about what to eat, let's talk about *how* to eat to lose weight. To begin with, the body likes its old habits. It grumbles and complains when something is changed. After previously eating a lot to satisfy your hidden hunger (no doubt the cause of your overweight) you are now going to eat less. You will soon adjust to eating less, because it is going to contain more value and less bulk. This will satisfy your needs and eventually your appetite. But not at first. Your stomach has been used to more food and it is going to continue to demand the same amount. It has become stretched to accommodate that large amount of bulk, and it is not going to give up without a struggle. The first three days on less food are the hardest. Shrinking your stomach is not easy. But it's like shrinking a balloon; once you shrink it, don't blow it up again. There are ways to appease your appetite while you are cutting the demands of your stomach.

Don't let yourself get too hungry. Fat has a lasting effect on hunger. Take a tablespoon of peanut butter or stuff a stalk of celery with it. You will be surprised how long the effect will last before you become hungry once more. Or, if you find yourself becoming shaky, irritable and weak, take a tablespoon or more of brewer's yeast in liquid. It is loaded with vitamins, minerals, and amino acids (protein factors) and will give you some lasting energy as well as appease your appetite. *Don't fall back on coffee without eating some protein with it.* It will only make you more irritable, more shaky and hungrier. Coffee encourages low blood sugar or hypoglycemia. It

95

gives you a quick pick-up but it is followed by a quicker let-down, making you want more and more coffee. The secret is to take some fat (peanut butter) or protein in some form, such as sunflower seeds or cheese, with your coffee, if you can't resist it. Or try a drink made with one of the many protein powders. This type of energy-lift lasts and also appeases hunger. Coffee does not.

After the three days are over, your stomach will stop pushing you. It gives up and lets you be the boss. But watch out for those Thanksgiving dinners and other feasts. They stretch the old stomach to large proportions again and you will have to go through three days of self-discipline all over again. It is really not worth it. You can eat, but merely eat less. The minute you feel full, stop! That childhood advice of "clean up your plate" does not apply to reducers.

Most overweight people are gulpers. They wolf their food and scarcely realize or even taste what they are eating. Many of them eat standing up, or eat and run. You would be surprised at how much food can be consumed this way without your even realizing it.

One movie star moved to Paris and suddenly realized she no longer had to fight the battle of the bulge. Others, who have spent time in France, say the same thing. They eat royally without gaining an ounce. The movie star discovered why. She says, "I don't gain weight in Paris. We eat slowly and our portions are not large. People in America eat on the run. Also, in Paris we don't have sweets and we eat our most important meal in the middle of the day which gives us a chance to work it off. Those large, late dinners are weight boosters."

This star has touched on several success secrets for reducing. The University of Chicago conducted a study which shows that a heavy meal at night does cause a weight gain. Your body uses up its fuel while you are expending a normal amount of energy during the day, but when you go to bed the process is slowed. Only a little fuel is needed while you sleep. The rest is stored as fat. Another woman gives her testimony about how this can lead to weight gain. She says that when she lived at home, the large meal, called "dinner" was eaten mid-day, and a light meal, called "supper" was eaten at night. She says that she did not have a weight problem. Later, she left home and ate her heavy meal at night. She soon began to gain. At first, she thought her metabolism was at fault until she returned home on a visit and returned to the old way of eating her heavy meal at noon. Her weight became normal without any dieting at all.

One reason why most people eat their heavy meal in the evening is that their families are away from home at lunch time and dinner is the occasion when the family can gather for a "square meal." More and more nutritionists and doctors are becoming convinced that the square meal should be breakfast, not dinner. The fuel eaten in the morning can carry a person through the day with far less fatigue. Grades are better for school children. Executives have less late morning slump. This means getting up earlier to enjoy a high protein meal of eggs with bacon or ham, plus fruit, instead of coffee, or juice and coffee, or juice, coffee and toast, eaten on the run. One child was found to be lethargic at school. He could not concentrate; his spirits were low and he was depressed. His teacher finally learned he had come to school without any breakfast at all because his family never had time to fix it or eat it. On inquiring further, she found there were other children with similar breakfast patterns. When these were corrected, either at home or at school, energy, enthusiasm and grades rose unbelievably. An engine without fuel cannot run far or well. This applies to cars, children, husbands and wives.

Many people say, "I *can't* eat a big breakfast. I am never hungry in the morning!" Adelle Davis has an answer to that one. She says the reason you aren't hungry in the morning is because you ate too much the night before. Her advice is, "Eat breakfast like a King, lunch like a Prince, and dinner like a pauper." It make take some replanning, but it can be done. If nothing else is possible, fix yourself and your family a high protein drink and let them *drink* their breakfast. Adding any of the protein powders available at health stores, to juice, plus a tablespoon or so of vegetable oil (you can't detect it) all whipped up in the blender can keep you going for hours and help maintain your weight, too.

I have been in Adelle Davis' home at breakfast time and watched her get her children off to school. Like all children, they were in a hurry, but she made such a nourishing drink, which her son named "Tiger's Milk," that they drank it before they left the house, or else! They really didn't mind because it is delicious. I know, since I had some, too. Adelle makes it of brewer's yeast, grated pineapple, canned or fresh, vanilla, all added to raw certified milk and mixed in a blender. It takes seconds to make, minutes to drink, and the effect lasts for hours.

There is another problem to watch out for: low blood sugar or hypoglycemia. It is becoming more and more common and doctors are finally getting around to recognizing it. It can cause shakiness, weakness, irritability, even blackouts. You may have been raised on the strict rule not to eat between meals. Today, this is actually dangerous. In many families, just before dinner, the children start squabbling, even the pets start fighting, and let's not discuss what goes on between husbands and wives who are ready to blow their tops. The whole thing may be because of low blood sugar due to the fact that the adults have not had anything since lunch, except a prolonged coffee break, and the children may have spent part of their lunch money (often unknown to parents) on a candy bar after school. Carbohydrates, candy and coffee merely perpetuate low blood sugar, whereas protein snacks such as cheese, sunflower seeds, and sprouts keep low blood sugar at bay. People *should* eat between meals and it should be something other than sweets (or coffee for adults). Sugar does not cure low blood sugar; it makes it worse. Protein helps control it. This newer knowledge of eating the right things oftener, not only keeps everybody feeling stronger and more cheerful, it also encourages weight loss. It is called the nibble diet.

The nibble diet is based on the premise that you spread out the amount of food you usually eat throughout the day but eat it oftener, not all at once in three "squares." Tests have proved that those who eat big meals are more overweight than those who ate 5 or 6 small meals a day, even though they had consumed no more food than usual. The nibble diet of small frequent meals is a beautiful way to shrink your stomach. Laboratory tests have shown that it is also helpful for avoiding high cholesterol, low blood sugar (hypoglycemia), heart disease and obesity. Less strain is put on the digestion by eating less at a time. By dividing up your food you can eat oftener, or whenever you wish, providing you don't eat junk. Don't even buy junk foods! If you see potato chips or candy or other sweets, when you look on the pantry shelf, you will eat it naturally. So will your children. But if it isn't there, you or they can't be tempted. Buy sensible food, or none. It is that easy. Ask your family for preferences, if you wish, both to give you ideas as well as to enlist their cooperation.

Mrs. Leanne E. Cupp of the Future Homemakers of America estimates that teen-agers eat at least one-fourth of their daily food in snacks. "There is gum and candy all morning, cookies and potato chips in the afternoon, a sandwich, cake and soda at home after school, and soda and pretzels with homework or TV after dinner—all 'empty calories.' "

Ben Weider, once writing in a health magazine, told how the nibble diet helped him. He says, "Try the nibble diet for yourself for one week. See how it works for you. Concentrate on high-protein foods, such as lean meats, fish, poultry, eggs, and milk. Then supplement these with low-carbohydrate vegetables such as broccoli, spinach, asparagus, celery, and lettuce. Be sure to eat a little fresh fruit every day and keep your bread down to a minimum, eating, all-in-all, only very small amounts of food several times during the day. *"Eat only until you are no longer hungry and no more!"* This may take quite a bit of self-training, since you have been eating on the three-meal plan for your entire life, and probably more than half the food you consume is eaten not to satisfy hunger, but merely out of habit.

"I have been on this diet myself for the past 10 days and have found everything wonderfully satisfying. I eat raw vegetables much of the time, and cold chicken or turkey every other day. At supper time I eat a hot meal, along with the rest of the family—but I eat *very, very little of everything.*

"Best of all, I have lost 4 pounds in these last 10 days, and I have never once felt the pangs of hunger!"

For those who can't work the nibble diet into their schedules, due to being away from home, there is still a way to eat, prevent hunger and lose weight.

Elizabeth Keyes, the founder of Overweight Over-comers International, has devised a method of losing weight which is unique, melts away the pounds without effort and delights those who have adopted it. Mrs. Keyes has written an enchanting little book explaining the process. It is called, *How to Win the Losing Fight* (available only from Gentle Living Publications, 2168 S. Lafayette, Denver, Colorado 80210). The book tells the whole story; I will merely give you an idea of how it works.

In general, Mrs. Keyes says, the method is based on the fact that all overweight people are gulpers. They swallow their food whole and, not being satisfied, take one helping after another. Here is her method: Take a bite the size of a pea. Put your fork down and relax while you chew it. Savor and enjoy every shred of flavor in that bite. When the bite has literally melted away in your mouth, then, and only then, take another bite and repeat the process. You will be amazed at how soon your appetite will disappear and how little food you will have eaten.

She tells of a woman who tried it. This woman was brought to a demonstration breakfast attended by fifty women, members of OOI. The overweight woman was evidently dragged there by a determined relative who wanted her to reduce. Mrs. Overweight was greeted by Mrs. Keyes and told she could order anything, absolutely anything, she wished for her breakfast. Defiantly she ordered hot cakes and syrup, butter, bacon and eggs, coffee with cream and sugar. When it was served to her, she fell to with gusto.

Mrs. Keyes said, "Wait! Cut off only a small bite, like this."

The woman complained, "I can't even taste that. It's so tiny I wouldn't know when I swallowed it."

But she followed directions. She held it in her mouth, tasted it, sucked the flavor between tongue and palate, closed her eyes, and enjoyed it to the fullest.

Mrs. Keyes then turned her attention to others around the table. She said, "After a while I noticed that my lady was sitting back, staring at her plate with a strange expression. She had eaten less than one-fourth of the cakes, one half-slice of the four slices of bacon, and had not touched the eggs.

" 'Is something wrong?' I asked.

"She shoved the plate back. 'Yes. It doesn't taste like I thought it would. In fact, it tastes awful. I've never been so disappointed in my life.' "

Mrs. Keyes coaxed her to take a little more. The woman said, "I don't want any more of the stuff. It would make me sick if I had to eat it."

Laughter went around the table as the other women cried, "She's converted."

Later that day the woman stopped Mrs. Keyes on the street. She said, "Do you know, I'm not hungry *yet*. Do you suppose something is wrong with me?"

Mrs. Keyes assured her that for the first time in years she was on the right track.

This woman, of course, was eating carbohydrates, as so many overweights do. By combining this method of eating to insure good assimilation, preventing gulping, and following the low carbohydrate-good nutrition diet, you have it made.

Does this mean that you can't ever go on binges? Be my guest! One physician says you can go on a binge now and then and still stay slim. However, as one drink leads to another, one binge leads to another until you are again living on binges. If you have satisfied your hidden hunger, the chances are that your craving for the things you used to eat will be psychological, only. You may feel sorry for yourself, wish to reward or pamper yourself, but the food you used to eat won't taste as good as you expected. You will usually find that that delectable lemon chiffon pie or chocolate cake, or even fluffy hot rolls are disappointing. So eat a bite or so and leave the rest. Or, if you are thumbing through magazines and see a picture of an Italian dinner, and think, "I simply *have* to have a spaghetti dinner complete with red wine," by all means have it! You will find it easier to live with yourself and others will find you easier to live with, if you yield to a binge now and then, say once a month. After all, it isn't so much what you eat, but how much. But remember, *the minute you feel full, stop.* Otherwise you will expand your stomach, again.

And before you yield to the next binge, look at yourself in the mirror. Which is more important, your new figure, or the binge? If you are willing to pay the piper and start the reducing, stomach shrinking, all over again, you are the one to make the choice, not I. So don't blame me if you gain back some of those hard lost pounds. As I said before, it is much easier to keep it off, than take it off.

Chapter 11

Are You a Water Storer?

What appears to be overweight is often nothing more than water retention. In other words, it is *water,* not *fat,* which may raise the pointer on the scales. You may be a chronic water storer, a problem which can be solved, as I will explain shortly; or you may start to retain water, without realizing it, as you begin your reducing program. One physician who specializes in weight loss problems says, "On a reducing diet the loss of weight occurs in a staircase pattern. First, excess body fat is burned. About four and one-half ounces of water are formed and stored within the tissues for every ounce of burned fat. Thus the dieter may not lose weight immediately; in fact he may gain several pounds for a brief period. But soon there is a change in the water tissue balance. The excess fluid is eliminated, and the scales show a weight loss."

This explains why, when you are reducing, you may reach a temporary plateau in your weight loss. This is also why some reducing specialists urge you not to weigh more often than once a week. They are afraid you will give in to discouragement. The weighing plan for the low carbohydrate diet, however, is a daily one. It is best to weigh at the same time daily, probably in the morning after going to the bathroom, without any clothing, and before eating or drinking anything. If you understand why these plateaus occur, you will not become unduly distressed.

Another physician explains, "Water is produced as fat is burned. In addition to what you drink, 1¼ pounds of water are produced in your body. This is nature's compensation to the body, but it can be mighty discouraging to the dieter."

Some doctors prescribe diuretics, but this can be hazardous. I remember being told what happened to a woman who checked into a "reducing farm" operated by a physician. In addition to being required to live on "rabbit food" only—carrots, celery, and the like—which kept her ravenous, the doctor gave her a strong diuretic tablet the first night after her arrival. The woman lost *nine pounds in one night,* during which she raced to the bathroom again and again. When morning came she was so weak from this sudden loss of weight she could scarcely move. But it was not only water which she lost, but vitamins. The vitamins B and C are water soluble, and such an excessive loss of water caused by the diuretic drugs carry these valuable vitamins out of the body. The woman stuck out her week at the reducing farm and returned home thinner, but weaker as well as wan. She could scarcely wait to get inside her own front door to start eating again. Within two weeks her weight was right back where it had been before her rugged experience at the reducing farm. She had not only parted with many pounds, which returned, but a lot of money, which didn't.

On a high protein, low carbohydrate diet with some fat, the weight loss would have been slower, but there would have been no weakness, nor ravenous hunger. The woman whom I later interviewed told me that the patients at that particular "resort" were a bundle of nerves, and no wonder! Vitamin B loss could account for part of this (vitamin B, together with calcium calms nerves) whereas the shock to the body of such sudden weight loss as well as continuous gnawing hunger could account for the rest. This is a kind of torture system from which dieters need not suffer.

Nutritional diuretics are safer, but before you try even them, you should understand what to expect from them and why. There is a water control mechanism built into your body. There are two minerals responsible for this control: sodium, which retains water, and potassium which eliminates it from the body. Many doctors, instead of prescribing drug diuretics, prescribe a low, or no sodium diet. They insist on your giving up salt, which contains sodium. For reducers, this is no good, because the body requires a certain amount of salt or sodium for health. What the doctors should do is to prescribe potassium instead, which will eliminate water. (Potassium tablets are available at health stores.) But still better, it is far wiser and more satisfactory in the long run, if you bring your own body's water control mechanism into balance. This can be done with a certain vitamin.

John M. Ellis, M.D., of Texas, in using vitamin B^6 successfully with his patients for nerve tingling and cramps in the calves of their legs, found that without changing their diet, these patients also began losing unnecessary weight, or inches. Cattlemen who rode the Texas range on large cattle ranches discovered they were able to tighten their belts to the last notch. And women who usually store water during pregnancy, menopause, or pre-menstrual periods, no longer suffered from this water storage problem. Many of Dr. Ellis' patients lost up to 3 inches in their waistlines, within a few short weeks. But when the vitamin B^6 was stopped, the good results also stopped.

Dr. Ellis was puzzled about this surprise effect of B^6 on water retention until he found the reason: vitamin B^6 apparently sets up a body balance of both sodium and potassium, which regulate the body fluids naturally. If you cut your sodium, or add potassium yourself, you may interfere with the correct water balance in your body. It is far wiser to let vitamin B^6 do it, naturally. And whenever you take any *single* B vitamin, you should always fortify it with a food high in *all* the B vitamin factors in natural, instead of synthetic form. Otherwise too much of one B vitamin can create a deficiency of another. Brewer's yeast, or liver (fresh or desiccated in tablets) are excellent sources of all the natural B vitamins.

Don't be afraid to eat salt while you are reducing, provided it is *whole sea or land salt,* guaranteed as such by the health food store. Remember, the usual salt found in supermarkets is sodium chloride only, which does influence water retention. Whole salt, whether from sea or land, contains all minerals, including sodium and potassium, which can help regulate your water balance. Don't avoid drinking water, either. Drink it whenever you are thirsty; it flushes away poisons and does not, by itself, cause water retention.

Therefore, while you are on your reducing, low carbohydrate diet, and suspect water retention, due either to weight loss or because you are a water storer, remember that vitamin B[6] plus a high powered food containing all B vitamins may speed results. Dr. Ellis' patients showed no side effects on taking 50 mg. of vitamin B[6] daily, even after three years. B[6] is available at health stores. After adding it to your diet, if your scales do not show a loss, try your tape measure. The body is working away trying to cooperate. Don't rush it. Eventually you should achieve success.

CHAPTER 12

Exercise, Smoking and Pitfalls

Exercise is really important if you want to reduce, stay healthy and firm. Every farmer knows that a well fed, unexercised animal becomes fat and flabby. This is one reason why city people walk their dogs. A well exercised dog or horse is sleek and firm. They also do not eat candies, cakes and pies or other carbohydrates or junk; nor do they drink alcohol. Animals are good examples of correct nutrition plus adequate exercise.

One reason that exercise is helpful is that it stirs up your circulation. It helps distribute the good nutrition you eat to all parts of your body, making you feel more alive and appear more attractive.

As people age, their circulation tends to slow down. Compare young people, who are rarely fat, to older people who are rarely thin. Young people are more active; elderly people are more sedentary. So exercise can make the difference because it helps to burn up the food which you eat so that it is not deposited as overweight. Unfortunately aging people become lazier, like aging animals, and usually don't exercise if they can help it. It seems to be too much effort and they don't enjoy it, anyway. This is probably because they aren't using the right kind of exercise for *them.*

Exercise can be as much a fad as clothes. At one time, setting up exercises were *the* thing. Then came jogging. Now it is Yoga. They are all helpful, providing you like them. You may prefer to swim, golf (without riding in a cart), play tennis, bowl, garden, or just walk, which is the best, easiest and cheapest of all. If you choose something you really like and set aside a particular time to do it, rather than waiting until you feel the urge, you can exercise daily with enjoyment. Also, stop pampering yourself. Don't ride when you can walk, or sit when you can stand. Activity and movement are preferable to remaining immobilized. They also burn up excess pounds.

Many housewives insist that they do not need to exercise because they get enough doing their housework. Housework is not the best type of exercise, although it may explain why women live longer than men. Nevertheless, the average housewife hates housework, and is resentful and tense all the time she is performing her chores. She also exercises the same old muscles day after day, leaving others untouched and fatigued because the circulation has not reached them. I proved this with a domestic who used to do my cleaning once a week. She arrived in the morning after a hectic race in getting her own house in order, her husband and children off to work and school. She admitted that she was exhausted before she even started on my house (and others whom she helped on other days). One day I asked her if she ever got any exercise. She looked at me as if I had lost my mind. "But that is all I do," she exploded. "I am on the move all the time."

I explained that it might be worth a try to do some relaxing exercise *other* than housework, and explained what I have already told you. She thought about it for awhile and then agreed to try it. The next week I scarcely recognized her. She told me that she had arranged to get up a little early and either take a refreshing walk before her family got up, or if that was impossible, she went through some exercises by an open window which reached and stretched all parts of her body. She told me that within three days she felt more alive and less fatigued. She also *wanted* to do those setting-up exercises to improve her figure, so she did not fight them every step of the way as she did housework, which she disliked, though she needed it for income.

This was a lesson for me, and I hope it will be for you. Choose something which really interests you, make it regular, and the improved circulation will increase your energy as well as reduce your weight. Spot exercises are fine, too. They firm up your tummy, cinch your waist, and stretch your back. Whether they are Yoga (which is excellent, providing you like it) or are taken from any one of hundreds of examples from books or TV programs, the secret of success is whether or not it suits *you*.

Smoking

Giving up smoking often causes people to gain weight. This is usually because they substitute eating for smoking. A well known nutritionist told me that she had finally given up smoking, but rewarded herself with some hard candy, which not only put on weight but increased her dentist bill due to the resulting cavities.

Smoking is a habit, as we all know, and as we also know, isn't good for you. It often is used as a tranquilizer against stress (vitamin B and calcium is better). It also represents the need for security and provides a crutch as well as the sucking motion of a baby who is using a pacifier. Whenever I see a man smoking a cigar, I think of the similarity. But smoking can also indicate low blood sugar. Smoking often indicates "hidden hunger," too. Smokers are seeking "something," they aren't sure what.

When people stop smoking, even if they do overeat and gain weight, this is usually only temporary. If one eats good nourishing food, as we have discussed in this book, the transition is easier. The body eventually adjusts, one feels better, and the metabolism improves, resulting in normal weight. The nibble diet may be a big help for those who are giving up smoking.

I will give you the steps in a new method which claims one can stop smoking and lose all desire to smoke. William P. Knowles, an English expert on breathing, says that of students from 100 countries, eight out of ten have stopped smoking entirely or greatly reduced their intake. A secretary, who smoked 25 cigarettes daily, suffered from bronchitis and a cough, stopped smoking in two months, after taking the course two years ago. Recently she tried a cigarette to test herself; the taste, she said, was awful. "My desire to smoke is gone, along with the bronchitis and the cough."

Here are the steps of the Knowles system. It is done three times daily, for three minutes each.*

1. Sit upright in a chair. Don't touch the back of the chair with your spine.

2. Stretch your arms forward, then draw them back slowly; let your elbows rest against the sides of your body; put hands—palms down—on your thighs.

3. Breathe in and out quickly through your nose about a dozen times. A smoker may cough and sputter, but this is good for expelling phlegm and stale air.

4. Once the lungs are cleansed, exhale slowly and completely until there is no air left in your lungs. Then inhale to the count of seven. Pause for one second, exhale. Do this breathing 14 times, seven in and seven out. Keep your chest out and shoulders back to allow freedom for breathing. That's it!

Restaurants

Maintaining your weight in restaurants is easy. You have no feeling of obligation to eat anything you don't want. By learning the rules and choosing foods according to your carbohydrate allowance, you can make it, providing you do not let your gaze wander toward the plates of others who are eating French fries, white buns, and other no-nos. If you must succumb, treat it as your monthly

---

*This was previously quoted in my question and answer column in *Let's Live* magazine, but it is well worth repeating.

binge, eat as little as possible, chew it as well as possible, and you will still survive.

Face Ravages

If you are losing weight, the first five pounds which come off, usually are noticeable in your tummy, and your face and neck. People may exclaim, "Don't you feel well?" You can prevent this kind of reaction if you do your face exercises as regularly as your body spot exercises. Your face has muscles and needs exercising, too. There are several face exercise books available to help you.

Stop Talking, Start Dieting

When you start dieting, keep it a secret. For some strange reason, if you tell people you are taking off some weight, they do everything in their power to stop you. I wish you would explain why, I can't. Your family will look at you in alarm, and tell you you don't need to lose weight. Your friends will warn you that you will fall apart. (On their diet, you may.) So button up your lip. You will get much further.

Stop thinking you are on a diet. You really aren't, you know; you are adopting a new way of life which incidentally will bring your weight under control and improve your health. Later, when everyone begins to clamor for your secret, you can tell them *then,* not before.

So keep up your vitamins, minerals, plus the low carbohydrate, high protein, medium fat diet. Get regular exercise. And most of all, give your subconscious some motivation. Every night as you drift off to sleep, make a picture of yourself as you wish to look: slender, healthy and radiant. Let the whole project become as automatic as driving your car. Once you have mastered the rules, and follow them, it will become second nature.

Spend your allowance of 60 grams of carbohydrate wisely.

CHAPTER 13

Check List for Drop-Outs

There are a few people who refuse to lose or are slower to lose on *any* reducing program.

Before you give up on this plan, which has succeeded where others have failed, check the following items. Those who have failed have later succeeded by correcting one or more possible pitfalls:

1. Are you *guessing* about the number of carbohydrate grams you eat? Don't! Only by tabulating them *every time you eat,* can you be sure. Total them at the end of the day. Guessing is the cause of many failures.

2. Overweights are gulpers. Chew everything to a pulp and savor the taste. Recently, at a business luncheon, the only overweight present had finished eating before the others had really begun.

3. Are you on a plateau? The body tries to compensate for any sudden change, often by storing water to maintain weight. If so, give it time. Some people have remained the same or even gained, though adhering faithfully to the gram count for a week or more. Eventually the weight loss occurred. Don't give in to discouragement.

One woman remained on a plateau after an initial weight loss and had about reached the conclusion that she would never lose any more. The next night, having made no changes in her diet or supplements, she visited the bathroom several times during the night. By morning the scales showed a substantial loss of weight without a feeling of weakness.

4. A *few* people need less carbohydrates than the 60 grams allotted. Every one is different, however, as you have seen. There is no rule without an exception. George

Watson, Ph.D., recently pointed out in his book, *Nutrition and Your Mind,* that there may be two types of eaters: fast oxidizers and slow oxidizers. (Oxidization is the speed at which a body breaks down its food in order to create energy). Dr. Watson believes that fast or slow oxidizers are not normal because their body chemistry is out of kilter. This might be the hidden factor which interferes with desired loss of weight. It may explain the situation of the couple I mentioned earlier, in which the wife remained a svelte size 8, although she actually ate more food than her husband who was 50 pounds overweight. She may be a fast oxidizer and he a slow one.

What are some of the differences between the two types? According to the Watson theory, a fast oxidizer, for example, may thrive on a big breakfast, whereas a slow oxidizer doesn't; he may feel worse afterward. A slow oxidizer seems to have more trouble breaking down his fat and protein foods, and often craves sour things. This is a giveaway that he may be short of hydrochloric acid and thus craves acid (and sometimes salt, which is needed for the manufacture of HCL). HCL definitely helps the breakdown and assimilation of protein.

According to Dr. Watson, the slow oxidizer may be able to eat more carbohydrates than fast oxidizers without disturbance. The picture of the fast versus the slow oxidizers is not yet clear, but it does remind us that we may differ in the way we break down our foods, even carbohydrates. One man, carefully watching his reactions, found he could eat only 30 grams of carbohydrates daily without side effects. He ate protein at each meal, took a full array of supplements, walked at least a mile a day, lost 33 pounds in six weeks with no hunger whatsoever, and said he felt wonderful. Several women have told me that they did not lose until they cut their carbohydrate grams to 50 grams daily and ate smaller helpings of food. But others may become weak if they cut back too far and this may be dangerous *for them.*

The body needs a certain amount of carbohydrate, so don't go overboard!

Even if you are out of kilter and fit into one of these groups now, correct nutrition may help correct the condition. A woman who decided she must be a slow oxidizer, immediately began improving her nutrition by adding high powered foods, a full array of natural vitamins and minerals as well as hydrochloric acid. She feels so much better that she is convinced she will become more normal in her food assimilation as well as more successful in controlling her weight problem within six months time.

5. How is *your* digestion? Are you storing bulk instead of digesting it? Tension can disrupt digestion. Do you need hydrochloric acid?

6. Try rearranging your eating. Substitute smaller, more frequent meals for three squares a day (though not consuming more food). Or shift your main meal to mid-day. Large meals, particularly at night before bedtime, are not used or digested, but stored as fat. Many have lost weight by doing nothing else than eating lightly at night.

7. Are you eating enough fat? As Ernest R. Reinsh, M.D., says, natural fat helps to burn up body fat and plays a prominent role in controlling obesity. Fat also supplies energy and staves off hunger.

8. Are you getting your full quota of vitamins and especially, minerals? Starved tissues often slow down weight loss. Also fill those tissues with good foods, not junk. They will crave less food.

9. If you tend to store water, are you taking vitamin B[6] daily, as suggested by John M. Ellis, M.D., who recommends 50 mg. of B[6] daily? The entire B complex in natural form should be added whenever a single B factor is used, to maintain correct balance in the B vitamin family. Otherwise, too much of one could cause the loss of another. Brewer's yeast or liver (desiccated if you prefer) are two good sources of the entire B complex. Watch

your alcohol intake, too. Alcohol burns up B vitamins and can encourage water storage.

10. Are you getting enough exercise? Exercise stimulates better circulation which helps your body to burn fat.

11. On your new program, if you are at a loss as to what to eat, and still cling to the old pattern, substitute a raw salad for a sandwich at lunch. If you are hurried or hate breakfast concoct a flavorsome protein drink. (Add protein powders from health stores to juice. Also add 2 tablespoons of oil. Mixed in a blender you will never know it's there.)

As a last resort, if you still do not lose, you can probably get off dead center by giving your body a jolt through a short version of one of the three detoxification diets mentioned in *Secrets of Health and Beauty*. These diets were not designed for reducers, per se, and should, in my opinion, not be continued longer than three days. On the fourth day you could drink juices and the fifth day eat raw salads before getting back on the low carbohydrate diet again. Vitamin and mineral supplements should be continued simultaneously. If you do continue the detoxification diet longer, you will become so hungry you may gain all lost weight immediately. This cleansing diet should not be repeated oftener than once a month, but could, through the loss of a few pounds, break the vicious cycle of no weight loss at all in a resisting body.

12. Finally, and this may be the greatest hitch of all: *do you really want to lose weight?* Many people insist they do, but they are actually overeating or mis-eating to compensate for some slight: lack of love or attention, resentment, hurt, or disappointment. Even if you are eating the right things and amount, you may be telling your subconscious you can't lose. Instead, give it orders three times a day to lose weight to help you look more attractive and feel better. Before going to sleep, visualize yourself looking and feeling slim. Pictures and feeling are the language the subconscious understands.

These extreme measures are only for the exceptions to successful weight losing on the low carbohydrate program. The majority responds with excellent success.

13. So set up your new program, eliminate your old faults, turn your attention away from eating to other things. Your new way of life will soon become automatic.

The Go, Stop, Caution Carbohydrate Computer

For the average person, the Carbohydrate Computer is the road map to a pleasant, hunger-free method of weight loss. William I. Kauffman, in the introduction to his little book, *The New Low Carbohydrate Diet,* states that you can lose 10 pounds in two weeks. Other carbohydrate counters promise a loss of from 3 to 5 pounds a week, or 10 to 15 pounds per month.

Mr. Kauffman states that he has been a weight watcher for twenty-five years, and that the low carbohydrate diet is the simplest, easiest way to lose weight he has ever known. He also assures us that the diet is satisfying, and hunger-free.

I have not listed any menus in this book for you. In general, try to have some protein, a little fat (oil or butter) and something raw with each meal. Most important, choose the 60 grams from the carbohydrates which help your health, not tear you down. I have listed all carbohydrates, good or bad, which appear in other carbohydrate counters, so you will learn to recognize which is which. But to help you choose the best ones, I have divided them into groups with names like traffic lights: GO, STOP, CAUTION. The GO carbohydrates are the higher powered foods, with extra nutrition, which help build up your health and vitality. The STOP group are empty calories only and do nothing for you. The CAUTION carbohydrates are in between, to be used with caution. Don't overdo them. You need not add anything for your daily quota for lecithin or vitamins or minerals. The count is minimal.

Keeping Score

First Week	Weight	Total Grams for Day
First Day		
Second Day		
Third Day		
Fourth Day		
Fifth Day		
Sixth Day		
Seventh Day		

Beginning Weight _____

End of Week Weight _____

Loss for One Week _____

GO-STOP-CAUTION
CARBOHYDRATE COMPUTER

ALPHABETICALLY ARRANGED
(ALCOHOLIC BEVERAGES AT END)

G = GO
S = STOP
C = CAUTION

A

	Grams			Grams
Abalone, broiled 3½ oz.	3.0 G	Apple juice (see juices)		
Abalone, canned, ⅔ C	2.9 G	Apple pie (see pies)		
Alcohol (separate list)		Apples		
Almonds		Raw, 1 large		27.3 G
In shell, 1 C	7.8 G	Raw, 1 medium		16.9 G
Shelled, ½ C	14.0 G	Raw, 1 small		11.1 G
Salted, 12 to 15	2.9 G	Raw, 1 C slices		19.0 G
Salted, chopped, 1 T	1.8 G	Baked, 2 T sugar, 1 large		51.3 C
Chocolate covered, 10 med.	16.9 S	Dehydrated (1 lb)		413.0 C
Ambrosia, ½ C	23.2 C	Dried (1 lb)		332.0 C
Anchovies, canned, 8 small fillets	trace G	Dried, cooked, unsw., 1 C		50.8 G
Anchovy paste, 1 t	.3 G	Dried, cooked, sw., 1 C		77.0 C
Apple brown betty (see puddings)		Frozen, sweet, ½ C slices		25.0 C
Apple butter, 1 T	8.5 C	Apples & apricots, canned, strained, 1 oz.		5.0 C
Apple cider (see cider)		Applesauce, canned, unsw., 1 C		26.2 G
Apple dumpling (see puddings)		Applesauce, canned, sw. 1 C		50.0 C

121

Food	Value
Applesauce, canned, strained, 1 oz.	5.5 C
Apricot nectar (see juices)	
Apricot pie (see pies)	
Apricots	
Fresh, 3 medium	13.0 G
Candied, 1 med.	26.0 S
Canned, 1 C with syrup	54.8 C
Canned, 4 halves, 2 T syrup	26.4 C
Canned, water pack, 1 C with liquid	19.8 C
Canned, low calorie, ½ C	9.2 C
Canned, strained, 1 oz.	9.8 C
Dried, 5 sm. halves	12.5 G
Dried, 1 C, 35-40 sm. halves	100.0 G
Dried, cooked, unsw., ½ C with liquid	31.1 G
Dried, cooked, sw., ½ C with liquid	51.4 C
Frozen, sw., ½ C	32.5 C
Arrowroot, 1 T	7.0 G
Artichoke hearts, canned, 5	8.0 G
Artichokes, French, 1	14.2 G
Artichokes, Jerusalem, 4 sm.	16.5 G
Artichokes, bottom, 1	5.0 G
Asparagus, 1 C cut spears	6.0 G
Asparagus, 6 stalks cooked	3.0 G
Asparagus, canned, 1 C cut spears	6.0 G
Asparagus, canned, 6 spears	3.4 G
Asparagus, frozen, 6 spears	3.9 G
Asparagus soup (see soups)	
Avocado, Calif., ½ medium	6.0 G
Avocado, Calif., 1 C cubes	9.0 G
Avocado, Florida, ½ medium	11.0 G
Avocado, Florida, 1 C cubes	13.0 G
B	
Bacon, broiled or fried, 1 lb.	4.8 G
Bacon, broiled or fried, 2 strips	.2 G
Bacon, Canadian, cooked, 1 slice	trace G
Bacon fat (see fats)	
Bagel, 1 med	32.5 S
Baked beans (see beans)	
Bamboo shoots, 1 C	7.9 G
Banana fritter, 1	11.4 S
Banana custard or whip (see puddings)	
Bananas	
Fresh, 1 large	44.4 G
Fresh, 1 medium	34.5 G
Fresh, 1 small	23.0 G
Fresh, 1 C slices	35.4 G
Fried in butter, 1 med.	34.6 G
Barley, dry, 1 C	160.0 G
Bass, baked	.0 G
Bass, broiled	.0 G
Bass, canned	.0 G
Bavarian cream (see puddings)	

Food	Value
Bean curd, 1 portion	2.4 G
Bean soup (see soups)	
Bean sprouts, mung, cooked, 1 C, drained	5.2 G
Bean sprouts, raw, 1½ C approximate average	5.0 G
Bean sprouts, soy, cooked, 1 C, drained	3.7 G
Beans	
Baked, canned, pork & molasses, 1 C	54.0 C
Baked, canned, pork & tomato sauce, 1 C	43.1 C
Baked, canned, without pork, 1 C	52.2 C
Green, 1 C, cooked	6.0 G
Green, canned, 1 C	9.6 G
Green, canned, strained, 1 oz.	1.1 G
Green, frozen, cut, 1 C	14.1 G
Green, frozen, French-style, 1 C	14.4 G
Kidney, 1 C, cooked	42.0 G
Lima, 1 C, cooked	29.2 G
Lima, canned, 1 C	29.4 G
Lima, dry, 1 C, cooked	48.0 G
Lima, frozen, 3½ oz.	17.6 G
Navy, dry, ½ C	61.6 C
Pinto, dry, ½ C	63.7 C
Red Mexican, dry, ½ C	63.7 C
Soy, dry, ½ C	36.6 G
Wax, 1 C, cooked	6.0 G
Wax, canned, 1 C	9.6 G
Wax, frozen, cut, 1 C	14.8 G
White marrow, dry, ½ C	61.6 C
Beef	
Boiled	.0 G
Brains (see brains)	
Braised or pot-roasted	.0 G
Brisket	.0 G
Chuck	.0 G
Corned	.0 G
Corned, hash (see hash)	
Dried, chipped	.0 G
Dried, chipped, creamed, ½ C	6.1 G
Flank	.0 G
Hamburger	.0 G
Heart (see heart)	
Kidneys (see kidneys)	
Liver (see liver)	
Plate	.0 G
Pot pie, frozen, 8 oz.	40.8 G
Potted	.0 G
Roast	.0 G
Round	.0 G
Rump	.0 G
Short ribs	.0 G
Steak	.0 G
Stewing	.0 G
Tongue, broiled, 3 oz.	.4 G
Tongue, potted, deviled, 1 T	.1 G
Beef hash (see hash)	

Beef suet	.0 G
Beef & veg. stew (see stew)	
Beer (under alcohol)	
Beet greens, 1 C, cooked	5.6 G
Beets	
Raw, 2	9.6 G
Cooked, 1 C	16.2 G
Canned, 1 C	17.9 G
Canned, strained, 1 oz.	2.4 G
Pickled, 1 C	20.0 G
Bell pepper (see peppers)	
Beverages (see individual listings)	
Biscuits, baking powder, 1 medium	19.8 C
Biscuits, baking powder, 1 small	14.0 C
Blackberries	
Fresh, 1 C	18.0 G
Canned, 1 C with syrup	45.6 C
Canned, water pack, 1 C with liquid	22.5 G
Canned, low calorie, 1 C	18.4 C
Blackberry jelly (see jelly)	
Blackberry pie (see pies)	
Blackstrap molasses (see syrups)	
Black-eyed peas (see cowpeas)	
Blancmange (see puddings)	
Blintzes, 1 small	12.9 C
Blueberries	
Fresh, 1 C	21.1 G
Canned, 1 C with syrup	60.0 C
Canned, water pack, 1 C with liquid	21.8 G
Canned, low calorie, 1 C	17.4 C
Frozen, sweetened, 1 C	37.2 C
Frozen, unsw., 3 oz.	22.0 G
Blueberry pie (see pies)	
Bluefish, broiled or baked	.0 G
Bluefish, fried in 1 T butter	.1 G
Bologna, all meat, 8 oz., about 8 slices	2.0 G
Bologna, all meat, ½" slice	.2 G
Bouillon (see soups)	
Bouillon cube, beef or chicken, 1 cube	.0 G
Bourbon (see alcohol)	
Boysenberries, frozen, sw., 1 C	35.2 C
Boysenberries, frozen, unsw., 1 C	11.8 G
Brains, all kinds, 3 oz.	.7 G
Bran flakes (see cereals)	
Brandy (see alcohol)	
Brazil nuts, 1 medium	.4 G
Brazil nuts, in shell, 10	4.8 G
Brazil nuts, shelled, ½ C	7.5 G
Bread crumbs, dry, 1 C	63.8 C-S
Bread crumbs, dry, 1 T	4.0 C-S
Bread pudding (see puddings)	
Bread stuffing (see stuffing)	
Breads	
Banana tea, 1 slice	21.8 S

Food	Value
Boston brown, ¾″ sl.	21.4 S
Bran, 1 sl.	17.0 C
Bran raisin, 1 sl.	27.2 C
Brown nut, 1 sl.	27.2 C
Cinnamon, 1 sl.	15.9 S
Corn, 1 sl.	21.1 C
Corn, southern style, 2″ square	21.6 C
Cracked wheat, 1 sl.	11.8 G
Date nut, 1 sl.	28.0 C
French, 1 lb.	236.1 S
French, 1 sm. slice	10.4 S
Ginger (see cakes)	
Gluten, 1 sl.	8.7 C
Graham, 1 lb.	220.0 G
Graham, 1 sl.	11.0 G
Italian, 1 lb.	243.8 S
Italian, 1 sm. slice	10.7 S
Melba toast (see toast)	
Protein, 1 slice	8.7 G
Pumpernickel, 1 lb.	237.9 G
Pumpernickel, 1 sl.	15.9 G
Raisin, 1 lb.	266.0 C
Raisin, 1 sl.	13.3 C
Roman meal, 1 sl.	13.7 G
Rye, light, 1 lb.	237.9 G
Rye, light, 1 sl.	12.1 G
Rye, dark, 1 sl.	15.9 G
Rye, party sliced, 1 sl.	7.9 G
Rye and wheat, 1 sl.	12.1 G
Short, 1 sl.	21.6 C
Spoon, 1 serving	17.0 G
Vienna, 1 lb.	236.1 C
Vienna, 1 sm. sl.	10.4 C
White, 1 lb.	235.2 S
White, 1 sl.	11.9 S
Whole wheat, 1 lb.	222.5 G
Whole wheat, 1 sl.	11.3 G
Whole wheat, raisin, 1 sl.	15.0 G
Zwieback (see toast)	
Breakfast foods (see cereals)	
Broccoli, 1 stalk	5.5 G
Broccoli, 1 C, cooked	8.2 G
Broccoli, frozen, 2-3 spears	4.3 G
Broccoli, frozen, chopped, ½ cup	4.6 G
Brown betty (see puddings)	
Brown sugar (see sugar)	
Brownies (see cookies)	
Brussels sprouts, 1 C, cooked	12.4 G
Brussels sprouts, frozen, 1 C	16.6 G
Buckwheat flour (see flour)	
Buckwheat pancakes (see pancakes)	
Buffalo meat	
Buns	.0 G
Cinnamon, 1	25.6 S

Cinnamon, raisin, 1	28.6	S
Hot cross, 1	20.0	S
Pecan, 1	37.0	S
Butter, 1 C	1.8	G
Butter, 1 T	.1	G
Butter, sweet, 1 T	.1	G
Butterfish, baked or broiled	.0	G
Buttermilk (see milk)		
Butternuts, 4 or 5	1.3	G
Butterscotch candy (see candies)		
Butterscotch sauce (see sauces)		

C

Cabbage, 1 C shredded	5.4	G
Cabbage, 1 C cooked	9.0	G
Cabbage, Chinese, 1 C	2.4	G
Cabbage, Chinese, 1 C cooked	4.6	G
Cabbage, cole slaw (see salads)		

Cakes

Almond coffee, 1 sl.	32.8	S
Angel food, 1 sl.	33.0	S
Apple crumb, 1 sl.	49.1	S
Applesauce, 1 piece	18.7	S
Butter, plain, 1 sq.	36.3	S
Butter, iced, 1 sq.	46.1	S
Caramel, iced, 1 sl.	44.1	S
Cheesecake, 1 piece	27.8	C
Cheesecake, pineapple, 1 piece	37.0	C
Chocolate, plain, 1 pc.	22.8	S
Chocolate, iced, 1 pc.	45.0	S
Chocolate layer cake, 1 piece	54.8	S
Coconut, iced, 1 piece	50.0	S
Coffee, plain, 1 piece	31.6	S
Coffee, iced, with nuts, 1 piece	32.8	S
Cup, plain, 1	22.8	S
Cup, iced, 1	31.0	S
Date torte, 1 serving	38.1	S
Fruit, 1 slice	22.4	C
Gingerbread, 1 square	26.9	S
Gold, 1 slice	14.8	S
Jelly roll, 1 slice	38.8	S
Layer, 2 layers, 1 pc.	54.4	S
Layer, 3 layers, 1 pc.	72.5	S
Marble, 1 slice	31.0	S
Pineapple upside-down, 1 piece	71.2	S
Pound, 1 slice	14.8	S
Shortcake (see shortcake)		
Sponge, 1 piece	21.8	S
Sunshine, 1 piece	36.3	S
Washington cream, 1 pc.	39.1	S
Calves' liver (see liver)		
Candied apricots (see apricots)		
Candied cherries (see cherries)		
Candied citron, 1 oz.	22.7	S

Food		
Candied ginger (see ginger root)		
Candied peel, 1 oz.	22.9	S
Candies		
Almond Joy, 10¢ size	21.8	S
Bon bon, 1	9.4	S
Brown sugar fudge, 1 pc.	22.9	S
Butterscotch, 1 oz.	24.3	S
Butterscotch, 1 pc.	4.3	S
Caramel, 1 oz.	22.0	S
Caramel, 1 med.	7.8	S
Caramel, chocolate nut, 1 piece	8.8	S
Chocolate, bitter, 1 oz. square	8.3	S
Chocolate, bitter, grated, 1 cup	41.5	S
Chocolate, milk, 1 oz.	15.9	S
Chocolate, milk, with almonds, 1 oz.	16.9	S
Chocolate, semisw., 1 oz.	17.5	S
Chocolate, sweet, 1 oz.	17.8	S
Chocolate almonds, 1 oz.	16.9	S
Chocolate bar, 2 oz. bar	32.4	S
Chocolate bar, with nuts, 1 oz.	16.9	S
Chocolate cherry, 1	8.6	S
Chocolate cream, 1 oz.	20.0	S
Chocolate cream, 1 med.	8.6	S
Chocolate-covered almonds, 6	8.5	S
Chocolate fudge, 1 pc.	23.7	S
Chocolate kisses, 1	2.2	S
Chocolate mint, 5¢ size	23.0	S
Chocolate mint, 3 sm.	21.6	S
Clark bar, 5¢ bar	21.6	S
Coconut cream, 1 sq.	20.0	S
Cream mint, 2 sm.	2.7	S
Date cream, 1 oz.	20.0	S
Divinity, 1 pc.	22.9	S
Fondant, 1 patty	10.0	S
Fruit drops, 3	9.9	S
Fudge, 1 piece	22.9	S
Fudge, with nuts, 1 oz.	17.5	S
Glazed fruit, 1 lg. pc.	8.1	S
Gum drops, 1 large or 8 sm.	8.6	S
Hard, 1 oz.	28.0	S
Hershey milk chocolate, 5¢ bar	15.9	S
Hershey milk chocolate, almonds, 5¢ bar	15.7	S
Jelly beans, 10	16.5	S
Lemon drops, 1	5.0	S
Lifesavers, fruit, 1 roll	35.0	S
Lifesavers, mint, 1 roll	30.0	S
Lollipop, 1 lg.	56.0	S
Lollipop, 1 med.	28.0	S
Maple sugar (see sugar)		
Mars bar, 1½ oz. bar	21.8	S
Mars Milky Way, 1 bar	58.3	S
Mars Three Musketeers, 1⅛ oz.	35.1	S
Marshmallow, 1 oz.	23.0	C
Marshmallow, 1	6.2	C

Food	Value	Food	Value
Marshmallow, chocolate, 1	8.5 S	Cooked, 1 C diced	9.4 G
Mints, after dinner, 5 sm.	1.3 S	Canned, 1 C diced	9.6 G
Mints, chocolate (see candies, ch. mint)		Canned, strained, 1 oz.	1.6 G
Molasses kisses, 1	6.0 S	Frozen, ½ C	4.6 G
Mounds, 10¢ bar	58.6 S	Casaba melon, 1 wedge	12.8 G
Nestle's milk chocolate, 5¢ bar	15.4 S	Cashew nuts, 1 C roasted	35.0 G
Nestle's milk chocolate, almonds, 5¢ bar	15.2 S	Cashew nuts, 1 oz.	8.3 G
Nestle's milk chocolate, crunch, 5¢ bar	15.0 S	Cashew nuts, 6 to 8	4.1 G
Nestle's semisw. bits, 1 oz.	16.8 S	Cassava, 3½ oz.	83.5 G
Oh Henry, 1 bar	21.8 S	Catfish	.0 G
Orange drops, 1	4.9 S	Catsup, 1 T	4.2 G
Peanut bar, 2 oz.	17.2 S-C	Cauliflower, 1 C buds, raw	4.9 G
Peanut brittle, 1 piece	20.6 S-C	Cauliflower, frozen, 1 C	7.6 G
Penny, 2 oz.	28.0 S	Caviar, 1 oz.	1.1 G
Snickers, 1 bar	25.1 S	Celeriac, 4 to 6 roots	8.8 G
Sourballs, 1	9.9 C	Celery, 1 large stalk	1.5 G
Cantaloupe, ½ melon	8.3 G	Celery, 1 C diced	3.7 G
Cantaloupe, 1 C diced	11.0 G	Celery, cooked, 1 C	4.8 G
Capers, 1 T	trace G	Cereals	
Caramel (see candies)		Bran, ¾ C	31.4 G
Caramel sauce (see sauces)		Bran flakes, ¾ C	22.6 G
Carbonated soft drinks (see soft drinks)		Cerevim, dry, ½ C	15.3 C
Carrot juice (see juices)		Cheerios, 1 C	17.7 S
Carrots		Corn, puffed, ¾ C	25.0 S
Raw, 1	5.1 G	Corn flakes, 1 C	21.0 S
Raw, grated, 1 C	10.2 G	Corn Flakes, sugar frosted, 1 C	35.0 S
Raw, sticks, 3	2.8 G	Corn grits, 1 C	26.6 S

Food		
Cream of Wheat, cooked, 1 C	26.8	S
Farina, cooked, 1 C	29.6	G
Grape Nuts, ¼ C	24.0	G
Grape Nut Flakes, ¾ C	23.0	S
Hominy, 1 C	26.6	C
Infant's dry, precooked, 1 oz.	20.4	C
Kellogg's Concentrate, ½ C	7.0	C
Kellogg's Special "K," 1 C	12.5	C
Kix, ¾ C	15.0	S
Krispies, ¾ C	25.1	S
Krumbles, ¾ C	23.8	S
Maltex. cooked, ¾ C	24.0	S
Maypo oat, cooked, ¾ C	21.0	S
Muffets, 1	18.2	S
Oat, ready to eat, 1 C	17.5	C
Oat, rolled, ⅔ C	17.3	G
Oatmeal, cooked, 1 C	26.0	G
Pablum, 2 T	4.3	S
Pep, 1 C	23.0	S
Post Toasties, ¾ C	15.0	S
Raisin Bran, 1 C	33.2	C
Ralston, cooked, ⅔ C	20.1	G
Ralston Wheat Chex, ¾ C	35.0	C
Rice, puffed, 1 C	11.7	S
Rice flakes, ¾ C	21.2	S
Rice Krispies, 1 C	25.1	S
Rolled oats, cooked, ⅓ C	19.3	G
Shredded wheat, 1 oz. biscuit	18.3	G
Sugar Krisps, 1 C	26.1	S
Wheat, puffed, 1 C	9.6	S
Wheat, puffed, sw., 1 oz.	17.6	S
Wheat, rolled, cooked, ½ C	20.0	G
Wheat & malted barley, cooked, ¾ C	21.7	G
Wheat flakes, 1 C	23.0	G
Wheatena, cooked, ⅔ C	21.0	G
Wheaties, 1 C	23.0	C
Whole meal, cooked, 1 C	40.0	G
Champagne (see alcohol)		
Chard, leaves, 1 C cooked	1.6	G
Chard, leaves & stalks, 1 C cooked	6.4	G
Cheese		
American, 1 oz.	.6	G
American, grated, 1 T	.1	G
Bleu, 1 oz.	.6	G
Blue, domestic, 1 oz.	.6	G
Brie, 1 oz.	.5	G
Camembert, 1 oz.	.5	G
Chateau, 1 oz.	1.1	G
Cheddar, 1 oz.	.6	G
Cheddar, grated, 1 T	.1	G
Cheddar, processed, 1 sl.	.6	G
Cheese food, 1 oz.	.3	G
Cottage, 1 C	4.5	G
Cottage, creamed, 1 C	5.7	G

Food	Value
Cream, 1 oz.	.6 G
Cream, 1 T	.3 G
Edam, 1 oz.	1.1 G
Feta, 1 oz.	.5 G
Gorgonzola, 1 oz.	.5 G
Gruyere, 1 oz.	.5 G
Liederkranz, 1 oz.	.6 G
Limburger, 1 oz.	.6 G
Mysost, 1 oz.	15.4 G
Neufchatel, 1 oz.	2.2 G
Pabst-ett, 1 oz.	2.2 G
Parmesan, 1 oz.	.7 G
Parmesan, grated, 1 T	.2 G
Pimiento, 1 oz.	1.9 G
Pot, 3 oz.	1.8 G
Provolone, 1 oz.	.8 G
Roquefort, 1 oz.	.5 G
Swiss, natural, 1 oz.	.5 C
Swiss, processed, 1 oz.	3.0 C
Velveeta, 1 oz.	10.8 G
Cheese fondue, 3½ oz.	
Cheese sauce (see sauces)	
Cheese souffle, ½ C	6.8 G
Cheese spreads (usually processed)	
Bacon, 1 oz.	1.9 C
Old English, 1 oz.	1.9 C
Olive pimiento, 1 oz.	1.9 C

Food	Value
Pimiento, 1 oz.	1.9 C
Pineapple, 1 oz.	2.9 C
Relish, 1 oz.	3.0 C
Roka bleu, 1 oz.	1.9 G
Cheese straws, 3	3.0 C
Cheesecake (see cakes)	
Cherries	
Fresh, sour or sweet,	14.8 G
15 large or 25 small	19.7 G
Fresh, pitted, 1 C	4.3 S
Candied, 1 large	22.0 G
Canned, Bing, low calorie, 1 C	59.0 S
Canned, Bing, in syrup, 1 C	23.8 G
Canned, red sour, water pack, 1 C	56.6 C
Canned, red sour, in syrup, 1 C	48.8 C
Canned, Royal Anne, in syrup, 1 C	21.0 G
Canned, Royal Anne, low calorie, 1 C	5.2 S
Maraschino, 1	7.2 G
Chestnuts, 2 large	
Chewing gum (see gum)	
Chicken	
Boiled	.0 G
Broiler	.0 G
Canned, boned	.0 G
Creamed, ½ C	5.7 G
Fryer	.0 G

Food	
Fryer, ½ bird, fried with butter and flour	6.2 G
Fryer, small leg, fried with flour	1.5 G
Gizzard	.0 G
Heart (see heart)	
Liver (see liver)	
Potted	.0 G
Roaster	.0 G
Stewing	.0 G
Chicken a la king, ½ C	6.6 C
Chicken broth (see soups)	
Chicken croquettes (see croquettes)	
Chicken fat (see fats)	
Chicken paprikash, small serving	5.7 G
Chicken pot pie, frozen, 8 oz.	50.4 C
Chicken salad (see salads)	
Chicken soup (see soups)	
Chicken TV dinner, 1	41.5 C
Chick-peas, ½ C, dry	64.0 C
Chicory, 10 sm. leaves	1.0 G
Chili con carne, ½ C, without beans	6.6 G
Chili con carne, ½ C, with beans	14.0 C
Chili powder, 1 T	.5 G
Chili sauce (see sauces)	
Chinese cabbage (see cabbage)	
Chipped beef (see beef)	
Chives, 1 T, chopped	trace G
Chocolate beverage, with milk, 1 C	17.1 S
Chocolate cake (see cakes)	
Chocolate candy (see candies)	
Chocolate ice cream (see ice cream)	
Chocolate malted (see milkshake)	
Chocolate milk (see milk)	
Chocolate milkshake (see milkshake)	
Chocolate pudding (see puddings)	
Chocolate sauce (see sauces)	
Chocolate syrup (see syrups)	6.6 C
Chop suey, with meat, canned, 1 C	9.6 G
Chow-chow (see pickles)	
Chow mein, chicken, canned, without noodles, 1 C	16.1 G
Chutney, apple, 5 T	52.3 C
Chutney, tomato, 5 T	38.8 C
Cider, fermented (see alcohol)	
Cider, sweet, 1 C	25.8 C
Cinnamon bun (see buns)	
Clam chowder (see soups)	
Cooked clam cocktail	
4 clams, 1 T sauce	4.5 G
Clam dip, sour cream, 3 t	.5 G
Clams (now considered polluted unless thoroughly cooked)	
Steamers, 6	4.4 G
Canned, 3 oz., drained	1.6 G

Food	Value		Food	Value
Canned, 3 oz., with liquid	2.2 G		Coffee with 1 T milk	1.5 C
Fried with batter, 6	9.5 C		Coffee with 1 T skim milk	1.6 C
Steamed, 6 with 1 T butter	4.6 G		Coffee with 1 t sugar	4.8 S
Stuffed, baked, 2	9.5 G		Coffee cake (see cakes)	
Club sandwich (see sandwiches)			Collards, ½ C, cooked	6.9 G
Coca Cola (see soft drinks)			Consommé (see soups)	
Cocoa, all milk, 1 C	24.8 S		Cookies	
Cocoa, ½ milk, ½ water, ¾ C	12.6 S		Animal crackers, 1	1.5 S
Cocoa, skim milk, ¾ C	17.2 S		Arrowroot, 1	3.6 S
Cocoa powder, 1 C	81.6 S		Brownies, 1	16.2 S
Cocoa powder, 1 T	5.0 S		Butter, 1	6.9 S
Cocoamalt, all milk, 1 C	33.5 S		Butterscotch, 1	14.6 S
Coconut, fresh, 2" sq.	6.3 G		Chocolate, 1	6.0 S
Coconut, fresh, shredded, 1 C	13.2 G		Chocolate chip, 1	7.8 S
Coconut, dried, shredded, sweetened, 1 C	33.0 C		Chocolate marshmallow, 1	8.6 S
			Chocolate wafer, 1	6.0 S
Coconut custard pie (see pies)			Coconut bar, 1	9.4 S
Coconut milk (see milk)			Date, 1	25.8 S
Codfish	.0 G		Devil's food squares, 1	11.8 S
Codfish, creamed, ½ C	8.1 G		Iced, 1	10.1 S
Codfish balls or cakes, 2	9.6 G		Fig bar, 1	11.4 S
Cod liver oil, 1 t	.0 G		Gaiety Creme Sandwich, 1	15.6 S
Coffee, black, 1 C	.8 C		Gingersnap, 1	3.2 S
Coffee with 1 T light cream	1.3 C		Gingersnap, 1 large	10.0 S
Coffee with 1 T evaporated milk	2.3 C		Graham cracker, 1	5.3 S
Coffee with 1 T heavy cream	1.2 C		Graham cracker, chocolate covered, 1	6.9 S
Coffee with 1 T condensed milk	11.1 C		Hermit, 1	6.9 S

Ladyfinger, 1	6.2 S
Lorna Doone, 1	5.4 S
Macaroon, 1	14.3 S
Molasses, 1	5.0 S
Nabisco, Devil, 1	11.8 S
Oatmeal, 1 large	17.0 S
Oreo Creme Sandwich, 1	8.7 S
Peanut, 1	7.3 S
Plain, 1 large	6.9 S
Raisin, 1	12.9 S
Scotch shortbread, 1	5.4 S
Social Tea, 1	3.8 S
Sugar	6.9 S
Sugar wafer, 1	1.5 S
Toll House, 1	7.2 S
Vanilla wafer, 1	3.6 S
Waffle creams, 1	7.2 S
Cooking fat (see fats)	
Corn, 1 ear	21.0 G
Corn, 1 C kernels	37.6 G
Corn, canned, 1 C kernels with liquid	51.2 G
Corn, frozen, ½ C kernels	17.6 G
Corn bread (see breads)	
Corn flakes (see cereals)	
Corn fritter, 1	10.2 C
Corn grits, ¼ C dry	28.4 G
Corn grits, 1 C cooked	26.6 G
Corn muffins (see muffins)	
Corn oil (see oils)	
Corn pudding, Southern, ½ C	13.4 C
Corn syrup (see syrups)	
Corned beef (see beef)	
Cornmeal, ¼ C dry, if undegerminated	28.9 G
Cornmeal, 1 C cooked, if undegerminated	25.5 G
Cornstarch, 1 T	7.0 S
Cornstarch pudding (see puddings)	
Cottage cheese (see cheese)	
Cowpeas, 1 C cooked	25.4 G
Crab, 1 lb. meat	2.3 G
Crab, canned, 8 oz.	2.5 G
Crab, deviled, 1 medium	9.7 G
Crab, soft-shell, fried with batter, 1 small	8.6 G
Crab apple, 1	3.5 G
Crab Jambalaya, 1 serv.	15.8 G
Crab paste, 1 T	.1 G
Crab salad (see salads)	
Cracker meal, 1 T	7.3 S
Crackers	
Animal (see cookies)	
Blue cheese, 1	1.4 G
Butter thins, 1	2.8 S
Cheese tidbits, 15 tiny	3.0 S
Graham (see cookies)	
Holland rusk (see toast)	

Item	Value		Item	Value
Matzoth, 1 6" piece	17.5 G		Sour, 1 C	7.7 G
Melba toast (see toast)			Whipped, ½ pint	3.6 G
Oyster, 10	7.1 S		Whipped, 1 T	.2 G
Peanut butter-cheese sandwich, 1	4.5 S		Cream cheese (see cheese)	
Pretzels (see pretzels)			Cream soup (see soups)	
Rice, Chico San	6.2 G		Crème de menthe (see alcohol)	
Ritz, 1	2.1 S		Creole sauce (see sauces)	
Rye thins, 1	1.9 C		Cress, garden, 1 lb.	15.0 G
Ry-Krisp, 1 dbl. sq.	9.6 C		Cress, garden, 1 C cooked	9.6 G
Saltine, 1	2.9 S		Cress, water, 1 lb.	15.2 G
Soda, 1	4.4 S		Cress, water, 1 bunch	3.3 G
Triscuit, 1	2.9 C		Cress, water, 10 sprigs	.5 G
Uneeda, 1	3.9 S		Crisco	.0 S
Water, 1	6.9 S		Croquettes, beef, 1 med.	8.8 S
Wheat, 1	4.4 G		Croquettes, chicken, 1 med.	8.8 G
Wheat thins, 1	1.3 G		Croquettes, fish, 1 med.	8.8 G
Zwieback (see toast)			Croquettes, potato, 1 med.	16.7 C
Cranberries, fresh, 1 C	10.8 G		Croutons, ½" cube	.6 C
Cranberry juice (see juices)			Cucumber pickles (see pickles)	
Cranberry relish, with orange, ¼ C	25.0 G		Cucumbers, 1 medium	2.8 G
Cranberry sauce (see sauces)			Cucumbers, 6 slices	1.4 G
Cream			Cupcake (see cakes)	
Light, ½ pint	8.2 G		Curaçao (see alcohol)	
Light, 1 T	.5 G		Currant jelly (see jams, jellies)	
Half and Half (see milk)			Currants, 1 C	17.0 G
Heavy, ½ pint	7.2 G		Currants, dried, sw., 1 C	142.4 G
Heavy, 1 T	.4 G		Curry powder, 1 T	.5 G

Custard (see puddings)
Custard pie (see pies)

D

Daiquiri (see alcohol)	
Dandelion greens, 1 lb.	40.0 G
Dandelion greens, ½ C cooked	8.0 G
Danish pastry (see pastries)	
Date torte (see cakes)	
Dates, 1 C pitted	134.0 G
Dates, 3 or 4	22.6 G
Deviled meat, 1 T	trace C
Dextromaltose, 1 T	6.8 S
Dill pickles (see pickles)	
Divinity (see candies)	
Doughnuts	
Cake, plain, 1	17.5 S
Cruller, sugared, 1	20.0 S
Jelly, 1	30.0 S
Raised or yeast, 1	13.7 S
Sugared or iced, 1	21.7 S
Dry milk (see milk)	
Duck	
Duck eggs (see eggs)	.0 G

E

Eclair (see pastries)	
Eels	
Eels, smoked	.0 G
Egg foo yung, 1 serving	.0 G
Egg roll, 1	6.5 G
Eggnog, alcoholic (see alcohol)	3.5 G
Eggnog, all milk, 1 C	24.7 G
Eggplant, ½ C	5.5 G
Eggplant, fried with batter, 1 slice	11.5 G
Eggs	
Raw, 1 medium	.3 G
Raw, whites, 1	.2 G
Raw, yolks, 1	.1 G
Boiled or poached, 1 medium	.3 G
Creamed, 2 eggs, 3 T sauce	5.1 G
Deviled, 1	.5 G
Dried, 1 T	.2 G
Dried, 1 C	2.7 G
Duck, 1 large	2.4 G
Fried, in butter, 1 medium	.4 G
Omelet, plain in butter, 1 egg	.4 G
Omelet, cheese, 2 eggs	.9 G
Omelet, Spanish, 2 eggs	7.6 G

Scrambled, with milk, 1 — 1.0 G
Endive, 2 stalks — 4.0 G
Endive, 10 inner leaves — 1.0 G
Escarole, 2 large leaves — 2.0 G
Escarole, 7 sm. leaves — .8 G

F

Fats
Bacon, 1 T — .0 C
Chicken — .0 G
Vegetable oil — .0 G
Fennel leaves, 2 pieces — 2.0 G
Fig bars (see cookies)
Figs
Fresh, 2 small — 19.6 G
Canned, 1 C with syrup — 79.6 C
Canned, low calorie, ½ C — 10.0 C
Dried, 1 C cut — 64.4 G
Dried, 1 large — 13.6 G
Kadota, 3, 1 T juice — 10.0 G
Filberts, 10 to 12 — 2.6 G
Finnan haddie — .0 G
Finnan haddie, creamed, 4 oz. — 6.1 G
Fish (see individual listings)
Fish, creamed, ½ C — 6.1 G
Fish cake (see cakes)
Fish cakes, 1 — 9.4 G

Fish croquettes (see croquettes)
Fish chowder (see soups)
Fish sticks, breaded, frozen, 4 oz. — 7.5 G
Flounder — .0 G
Flour
Buckwheat, 1 C — 70.6 G
Cake, 1 C — 72.2 S
Corn, 1 C, if undegerminated — 84.6 G
Rye, 1 C — 62.3 G
Soybean, 1 C — 38.1 G
Wheat, 1 C — 83.7 G
White, 1 C — 83.7 S
White, 1 T — 5.4 S
Fondant (see candies)
Frankfurters (contain additives),
1 cooked, about 1.8 oz. — 1.0 C
French bread (see breads)
French dressing (see salad dressings)
French pastry (see pastries)
French toast, without syrup, 1 piece — 12.2 S
French toast, 1 T corn syrup, 1 piece — 27.2 S
French toast, 1 T maple syrup, 1 piece — 25.0 S
Frog legs — .0 G
Frog legs, fried with batter, 2 — 4.0 G
Fruit (see individual listings)
Fruit cake (see cakes)
Fruit cocktail, fresh, 1 C — 34.2 G

Fruit cocktail, canned, 1 C with syrup — 47.6 C
Fruit cocktail, canned, low calorie, 1 C — 9.3 C
Fruit salad (see salads)
Fruits for salads, canned, low calorie, ⅔ C — 7.0 C
Fruits for salad, canned, 3 T — 29.0 C
Fruits, glazed (see candies)
Fudge (see candies)
Fudge sundae (see ice cream sundaes)

G

Garbanzos (see chick-peas)
Garden cress (see cress)
Garlic, 1 clove — .4 G
Gefilte fish, 4 oz. — 9.6 G
Gelatin, dry, plain, if added to protein — .0 G
Gelatin, fruit flavors, prepared, ½ C — 18.0 S
Gelatin, fruit flavors, fruit added, ½ C — 26.8 S
Gelatin salad (see salads)
Gin (see alcohol)
Ginger ale (see soft drinks)
Ginger root, 3½ C — 6.9 G
Ginger root, candied, 1 oz. — 24.7 S
Gingerbread (see cakes)
Gingersnaps (see cookies)
Glazed fruit (see candies)
Goat's milk (see milk)

Goose — .0 G
Gooseberries, 1 C — 12.9 G
Goulash, Hungarian, ½ C — 9.5 G
Graham crackers (see cookies)
Grape juice (see juices)
Grape Nuts (see cereals)
Grape soda (see soft drinks)
Grapefruit
  Fresh, ½ large — 22.2 G
  Fresh, ½ medium — 18.2 G
  Fresh, ½ small — 14.0 G
  Fresh, 1 C sections — 19.6 G
  Fresh, pink, ½ medium — 18.2 G
  Canned, 1 C with syrup — 42.6 S
  Canned, water pack, 1 C with liquid — 19.2 C
Grapefruit juice (see juices)
Grapes
  Fresh, American type (Concord, Delaware, Niagara), 1 C — 18.5 G
  Fresh, European type (Malaga, Muscat, Tokay), 1 C — 25.9 G
  Thompson seedless, ½ C — 16.7 G
  Canned, 1 C with syrup — 45.4 C
  Canned, water pack, 1 C — 22.0 G
Gravy, ¼ C thickened — 4.2 C
Green beans (see beans, green)
Green onions (see onions, green)

Item	
Green pea soup (see soups)	
Griddle cakes (see pancakes)	
Grits, hominy, ½ C cooked	13.3 G
Guava, 1	17.1 G
Guava butter (see jams, jellies)	
Guava jelly (see jams, jellies)	
Guinea hen	.0 G
Gum, chewing, 1 stick	1.7 S
Gum, chewing, candy coated, 2 pieces	2.5 S
Gumbo soup (see soups)	

H

Item	
Haddock	.0 G
Haddock, creamed, 4 oz.	6.1 G
Haddock, fried with flour, 1 fillet, about 3 oz.	8.1 G
Halibut, broiled	.0 G
Halibut, creamed, 4 oz.	6.1 G
Ham	
Fresh	.0 G
Baked, cured, 3 oz., no bone	.3 G
Boiled	.0 G
Canned, boneless, 3 oz.	.4 G
Canned, deviled, 1 T	.2 G
Canned, spiced, 2 oz.	.2 G
Prosciutto, 1½ oz.	.0 G
Smoked, cooked	.0 G
Ham sandwich (see sandwiches)	
Hamburger (see beef)	
Hamburger sandwich (see sandwiches)	
Hard candy (see candies)	
Hard sauce (see sauces)	
Hash, beef, 1 C	19.0 G
Hash, canned corned beef, with potatoes, 1 C	24.3 G
Hash, turkey, 1 C	19.0 G
Hazelnuts, 10 to 12	3.0 G
Head cheese, 3 oz.	.0 G
Heart, beef, lean, 3 oz.	.7 G
Heart, beef, braised, 3 oz.	.8 G
Heart, chicken, 3 oz.	1.3 G
Heart, pork. 3 oz.	.4 G
Herbs, 1 t	.0 G
Hermits (see cookies)	
Herring	
Atlantic	.0 G
Canned, in tomato sauce, 8 oz.	8.4 G
Lake	.0 G
Pacific	.0 G
Kippered	.0 G
Marinated with cream, small piece	.8 G
Pickled	.0 G

Smoked .0 C
Hershey bar (see candies)
Hickory nuts, 15 small 2.0 G
Highball (see alcohol)
Holland rusk (see toast)
Hollandaise (see sauces)
Hominy grits (see grits)
Honey (see syrups)
Honeydew melon, 1 wedge 12.8 G
Horseradish, 1 T .4 G
Hot dog (see sandwiches)
  (also see frankfurter)
Hubbard squash (see squash)
Huckleberries, 1 C 21.1 G

I

Ice cream
(regular commercial brands, not ice cream
sold in health food stores)
Plain, vanilla, ¼ pt. 15.1 S
Chocolate, ¼ pt. 16.6 S
Coffee, ¼ pt. 15.6 S
Frozen custard, ¼ pt. 16.3 S
Peach, ¼ pt. 15.9 S
Sherbet, with milk, ¼ pt. 44.0 S
Sherbet, with water (see ice cream, ices)

Strawberry, ¼ pt. 15.9 S
Ice cream, ices, ¼ pt. 35.2 S
Ice cream, milk, ¼ pt. 21.2 S
Ice cream cone (cone alone) 3.5 S
Ice cream parfait, coffee, 1 14.4 S
Ice cream parfait, maple, 1 19.9 S
Ice cream pop, chocolate covered 14.5 S
Ice pop, twin 23.7 S
Ice cream soda
Chocolate, vanilla ice cream, 10 oz. 47.9 S
Chocolate, chocolate ice
  cream, 10 oz. 48.7 S
Strawberry, strawberry ice
  cream, 10 oz. 48.2 S
Vanilla, vanilla ice cream, 10 oz. 47.1 S
Ice cream sundae
Banana split 92.5 S
Butterscotch 55.6 S
Chocolate (vanilla ice ceram) 52.8 S
Chocolate (chocolate ice cream) 54.3 S
Hot fudge 52.8 S
Ice, milk (see ice cream, milk)
Ice, water (see ice cream, ices)
Indian pudding (see puddings)
Irish whiskey (see alcohol)
Italian bread (see breads)

J

Jams, jellies

Blackberry jam, 1 T	14.2 S
Blackberry jelly, 1 T	13.0 S
Cranberry jelly, 1 T	8.6 S
Currant jelly, 1 T	13.0 S
Guava butter, 1 T	10.0 S
Guava jelly, 1 T	13.0 S
Grape jelly, 1 T	13.0 S
Lemon jelly, 1 T	13.0 S
Orange marmalade, 1 T	14.0 S
Papaya marmalade, 1 T	14.6 S
Plum jam, 1 T	14.2 S
Preserves, 1 T	14.2 S
Strawberry jam, 1 T	14.2 S

Jell-O (see gelatin)

Juices
(not fruit "drinks" which contain fillers)

Apple, fresh or canned, 1 C	34.2 G
Apricot, unsw., 1 C	29.2 G
Apricot nectar, 1 C	36.2 G
Blackberry, 1 C	18.0 G
Blueberry, 1 C	32.4 G
Carrot, 1 C	12.8 G
Cider (see cider)	
Cranberry, 1 C	36.0 G
Currant, black, 1 C	34.4 G
Currant, red, 1 C	25.2 G
Grape, 1 C	42.0 G
Grape, frozen, sw., 1 C	31.0 C
Grapefruit, 1 C	23.0 G
Grapefruit, canned, unsw., 1 C	24.0 G
Grapefruit, canned, sw., 1 C	30.4 C
Grapefruit, frozen, unsw., 6 oz. can	72.0 G
Grapefruit, frozen, sw., 6 oz. can	85.0 C
Grapefruit, frozen, sw., diluted, 1 C	28.0 C
Lemon, 1 C	18.9 G
Lemon, 1 T	1.2 G
Lime, 1 C	20.4 G
Lime, 1 T	1.2 G
Loganberry, 1 C	24.8 G
Nectarine, 1 C	34.9 G
Orange, California, Valencia, 1 C	27.0 G
Orange, Florida early season, 1 C	23.0 G
Orange, Florida late season, 1 C	27.0 G
Orange, canned, unsw., 1 C	27.0 G
Orange, canned, sw., 1 C	32.0 C
Orange, frozen, unsw., 6 oz. can	80.0 G
Orange, frozen, unsw., diluted, 1 C	24.4 G
Orange, dehydrated, 4 oz. crystals	100.0 G
Orange, dehydrated, water added, 1 C	24.7 G
Orange-grapefruit, canned, unsw., 1 C	23.6 G

Orange-grapefruit, canned, sw., 1 C	28.0 C
Orange-grapefruit, frozen, 6 oz. can	77.7 G
Orange-grapefruit, frozen, diluted, 1 C	24.0 G
Papaya, 1 C	30.2 G
Peach nectar, canned, 1 C	31.0 G
Pear nectar, canned, 1 C	32.0 G
Pineapple, frozen, unsw., 1 C	31.2 G
Pineapple, canned, 1 C	32.4 G
Pomegranate, 1 C	18.2 G
Prune, canned, 1 C	45.6 G
Raspberry, 1 C	25.6 G
Sauerkraut, 1 C	6.0 G
Tangerine, canned, sw., 1 C	27.0 C
Tangerine, canned, unsw., 1 C	25.0 G
Tangerine, frozen, 6 oz. can	80.0 G
Tomato, canned, 1 C	10.4 G
Vegetable, canned, 1 C	8.6 G
V-8, 1 C	8.6 G
Junket (see puddings)	

K

Kale, 1 C cooked	7.2 G
Kale, frozen, 3½ oz.	5.4 G
Kellogg's cereal (see cereals)	
Kidney beans (see beans)	

Kidneys	
Beef, ½ C	.9 G
Lamb, ½ C	1.0 G
Pork, ½ C	.8 G
Veal, ½ C	.9 G
Kippered herring (see herring)	
Kix (see cereals)	
Kohlrabi, ⅔ C diced	6.7 G
Kohlrabi, 1 C cooked	10.0 G
Kohlrabi, frozen, 1 C	10.4 G
Krispies (see cereals)	
Kumquats, 5 or 6	9.7 G

L

Ladyfingers (see cookies)	
Lamb	
Breast	.0 G
Chops	.0 G
Ground	.0 G
Kidney (see kidneys)	
Liver (see liver)	
Roast, leg	.0 G
Roast, shoulder	.0 G
Lamb curry, with rice, ½ C	22.9 G
Lamb shish kebab	.0 G

141

Food	Value
Lamb stew (see stew)	
Lambsquarter or pigweed, ½ C	8.3 G
Lard	.0 S
Layer cake (see cakes)	
Leeks, 3 medium	7.9 G
Lemon, 1 medium	8.4 G
Lemon drops (see candies)	
Lemon ice (see ice cream, ices)	
Lemon jelly (see jams, jellies)	
Lemon juice (see juices)	
Lemon peel, candied (see candied peel)	
Lemon pie (see pies)	
Lemon pudding (see puddings)	
Lemon sauce (see sauces)	
Lemon soda (see soft drinks)	
Lemonade, frozen conc., sw., 6 oz. can	112.0 C
Lemonade, frozen, sw., diluted, 1 C	28.0 C
Lentil soup (see soups)	
Lentils, ½ C	18.1 G
Lettuce, 1 compact head	13.0 G
Lettuce, 1 C	2.9 G
Lettuce, 4 sm. leaves	1.0 G
Lettuce and tomato salad (see salads)	
Lichee nuts, 6	10.5 G
Lichee nuts, dried, 3½ oz.	52.5 G
Liederkranz cheese (see cheese)	

Food	Value
Lifesavers (see candies)	
Limburger cheese (see cheese)	
Lime, 1 large	9.0 G
Lime juice (see juices)	
Limeade, frozen conc., 6 oz. can, sweetened	108.0 C
Limeade, frozen, diluted, sw., 1 C	27.0 C
Liquid diets, 1 day	110.1 C
Liver	
Beef, 3½ oz.	6.0 G
Calves', 3½ oz.	4.0 G
Canned, strained, 1 jar, 3½ oz.	1.8 G
Chicken, 3 oz.	3.0 G
Chicken, 1 med.	1.0 G
Chopped, 3 oz.	3.0 G
Goose, 2 medium	4.0 G
Goose liver paste (see Pâté de foie gras)	
Lamb, 1 slice	4.3 G
Pork, 1 slice	3.8 G
Liver loaf, 1 slice	9.4 G
Liver spread, 2 T	.2 G
Liverwurst, 1 slice	.5 G
Liverwurst sandwich (see sandwiches)	
Lobster	
Fresh, 1 lb. in shell	.6 G
Baked or broiled	.6 G
Broiled, 1 African tail, about ½ lb.	.3 G
Canned or cooked, ½ C	.7 G

142

Creamed, ½ C	6.4	G
Lobster Cantonese, 1 serv.	7.5	G
Lobster cocktail, ½ C meat, 2 T sauce	3.0	G
Lobster cocktail, ½ C meat, wedge lemon	.8	G
Lobster cocktail, ½ C meat, mayonnaise	.9	G
Lobster Newburgh, ½ C	7.7	G
Lobster paste, 1 t	.1	G
Lobster salad (see salads)		
Lobster Thermidor, 1 lobster	14.8	G
Loganberries, ⅔ C	15.0	G
Loganberries, canned, 1 C	25.0	G
Loganberry juice (see juices)		
Lollipops (see candies)		
Lotus root, ⅔ average segment	15.7	G
Lox	.0	G
Luncheon meat, 1 oz.	.5	G
Luncheon meat sandwich (see sandwiches)		
M		
Macadamia nuts, 10 to 12	1.5	G
Macaroni, cooked, 8-10 min., 1 C	39.0	S
Macaroni, cooked till tender, 1 C	32.0	S
Macaroni and cheese, 1 C	44.0	C
Macaroni salad (see salads)		
Macaroons (see cookies)		
Mackerel	.0	G

Madeira wine (see alcohol)		
Malted milk (see milkshake)		
Malted milk powder, 1 T	6.8	G
Maltex cereal (see cereals)		
Mandarin orange (see tangerines)		
Mango, 1 medium	34.5	G
Manhattan cocktail (see alcohol)		
Maple syrup (see syrups)		
Margarine, 1 C	1.8	G
Margarine, 1 T	.1	G
Margarine, 1 pat	trace	G
Marmalade (see jams, jellies)		
Mars candy (see candies)		
Marshmallow (see candies)		
Marshmallow sauce (see sauces)		
Martini cocktail (see alcohol)		
Mashed potatoes (see potatoes)		
Matzoth (see crackers)		
Mayonnaise (see salad dressing)		
Maypo oat cereal (see cereals)		
Meal, cracker (see cracker meal)		
Meat (see individual listings)		
Meat croquette (see croquettes, beef)		
Meat gravy (see gravy)		
Meat loaf, beef-pork, 1 sl.	11.5	G
Meat stew (see stew)		
Melba toast (see toast)		

Melon balls, frozen, 1 C	12.5 G
Melons (see individual listings)	
Meringue, ¼ C	8.3 S
Milk	
Whole, 1 C	11.8 G
Whole, 1 T	.7 G
Skim, nonfat, 1 C	13.0 C
Buttermilk, 1 C	12.4 G
Canned, evaporated, 1 C	24.0 G
Canned, evaporated, 1 T	1.5 G
Canned, sw. cond., 1 C	170.0 S
Canned, sw. cond., 1 T	10.3 S
Chocolate flavored, 1 C	27.9 S
Chocolate flavored, skim, 1 C	28.1 S
Cocoa (see cocoa)	
Coconut, 1 C	12.0 G
Dry, whole, 1 C	39.0 G
Dry, whole, 1 T	2.4 G
Dry, nonfat, 1 C	42.0 C
Dry, nonfat, 1 T	2.7 C
Goat's, 1 C	11.2 G
Half and half, 1 C	11.0 G
Malted (see milkshake)	
Milkshake, chocolate, 10 oz.	57.0 S
Milkshake, chocolate malted, 10 oz.	70.0 S
Mincemeat pie (see pies)	
Mineral oil (see oils)	
Mint, 1 t chopped	.0 G
Mint julep (see alcohol)	
Mints (see candies)	
Mixed vegetables (see vegetables, mixed)	
Molasses (see syrups)	
Muffins	
Blueberry, 1 small	23.2 S
Bran, 1 medium	20.5 C
Corn, 1 medium, if undegerminated	18.0 C
Date, 1 medium	40.8 C
Egg, 1 medium	20.2 C
English, 1 medium	17.5 C
Raisin, 1 medium	27.2 C
Soy, 1 medium	16.7 G
White, 1 medium	17.1 S
Whole wheat, 1 medium	17.1 G
Muscatel wine (see alcohol)	
Mushroom soup (see soups)	
Mushrooms, raw, ½ lb.	9.7 G
Mushrooms, raw, 4 large or 10 medium	4.0 G
Mushrooms, canned, 1 C with liquid	9.0 G
Mushrooms, sauteed, 7 sm.	2.8 G
Muskmelon, ½ medium	8.3 G
Mussels, 1 lb., if thoroughly cooked	7.2 G
Mussels, smoked, 1	trace C
Mustard, dry	.0 G
Mustard, prepared, 1 T	.8 G

Mustard greens, 1 lb.	13.2 G
Mustard greens, 1 C cooked	5.8 G
Mutton	.0 G

N

Nabisco wafers (see cookies)	
Navy beans (see beans, navy)	
Nectar (see juices)	
Nectarines, 2 medium	16.0 G
Noodle soup (see soups)	
Noodles, egg, 1 C cooked	37.0 C
Noodles, fried, canned, 1 oz.	16.7 C
Nuts (see inavivaual listings)	
Nuts, mixed, 8 to 12	2.7 G

O

Oatmeal (see cereals)	
Oatmeal cookies (see cookies)	
Ocean perch (see perch)	
Oils	
Corn	.0 G
Cottonseed	.0 S
Mineral (dangerous)	.0 G
Olive	.0 G
Peanut	.0 G
Safflower	.0 G

145

Salad	.0 G
Sesame	.0 G
Sunflower	.0 G
Okra, 8 pods cooked	6.3 G
Oleomargarine (see margarine)	
Olive cheese spread (see cheese spreads)	
Olive oil (see oils)	
Olives, green, 10 large	1.0 G
Olives, ripe or black, 10 lg.	2.0 G
Omelet (see eggs)	
Onion soup (see soups)	
Onions	
Raw, 1 medium	10.5 G
Raw, 1 T chopped	1.0 G
Cooked, 1 C	18.0 G
Dehydrated, 2 T	8.0 G
Green, 6 small	5.3 G
Scalloped, ½ C	15.2 G
Orange ice (see ice cream, ices)	
Orange juice (see juices)	
Orange soda (see soft drinks)	
Oranges	
Fresh, 1 large	26.0 G
Fresh, 1 medium	17.0 G
Fresh, 1 small	11.5 G
Fresh, 1 C sections	22.0 G
Ovaltine, 1 C	21.7 C

Food	Value
Oysters (if thoroughly cooked)	
Stew, 1 C, 6-8 medium	11.0 C
Stew, frozen, 1 can	19.6 C
Raw, meat only, 5-8 (considered polluted)	
Fried with batter, 6	5.6 C
Scalloped, 6	18.2 C
	31.6 C

P

Food	Value
Pablum (see cereals)	
Pancakes, buckwheat, 1 4'' cake	10.7 C
Pancakes, white flour, 1 4'' cake	12.9 S
Papaya, 1 C cubes	18.0 G
Papaya juice (see juices)	
Parfait (see ice cream parfait)	
Parmesan cheese (see cheeses)	
Parsley, 1 T chopped	.2 G
Parsnips, ½ C cooked	10.8 G
Passion fruit, ½ C	14.0 G
Pasta (see individual listings)	
Pastrami	.0 G
Pastries	
Cream puff, 1	15.7 S
Danish, 1 medium	22.8 S
Doughnuts (see doughnuts)	
Eclair, chocolate, custard, 1	20.3 S
Eclair, chocolate, cream, 1	15.7 S
French pastry, medium	15.0 to 40.0 S
Petit Fours, 1	25.0 S
Pâté de foie gras, 1 T	.7 G
Pea soup (see soups)	
Peaches	
Fresh, 1 medium	9.7 G
Fresh, 1 C slices	16.0 G
Canned, 1 C with syrup	49.0 C
Canned, water pack, 1 C with liquid	17.0 G
Canned, strained, 1 oz.	5.0 G
Dried, 1 C	109.0 G
Dried, cooked, unsw., 1 C with liquid	58.0 G
Dried, cooked, sw., 1 C with liquid	94.0 C
Frozen, sliced, sw., 1 C	56.0 C
Peanut brittle (see candies)	
Peanut butter, 1 T	3.4 G
Peanut butter, added to 1 stalk celery	4.9 G
Peanut butter sandwich (see sandwiches)	
Peanuts, 1 C halves	34.0 G
Peanuts, 18 to 20	4.2 G
Peanuts, 1 T chopped	2.1 G
Pears	
Fresh, 1	23.9 G
Fresh, 1 C quarters	31.8 G
Canned, 1 C with syrup	49.2 C
Canned, 2 halves with 2 T syrup	23.0 C

Canned, water pack, 1 C with liquid	19.8 G
Canned, low calorie, 1 C	14.4 C
Canned, strained, 1 oz.	4.5 G
Peas	
Fresh, 1 C cooked	19.0 G
Fresh, 1 pound, in pod	36.1 G
Canned, 1 C with liquid	32.2 G
Canned, 1 C, drained	27.6 G
Canned, strained, 1 oz.	2.0 G
Dried, ½ C cooked	18.1 G
Frozen, ½ C	11.3 G
Split, 1 C cooked	45.0 G
Peas, edible pods (see snow peas)	
Pecans, 12 nutmeats	1.8 G
Pecans, chopped, 1 T	.9 G
Pecans, 1 C halves	14.6 G
Pepperpot soup (see soups)	
Peppers, green, 1 medium	3.0 G
Peppers, green, chopped, 1 T	.5 G
Peppers, green, stuffed, 1 medium	12.2 G
Peppers, red, hot dried, 1 T	9.0 G
Peppers, red, 1 medium	4.0 G
Pepsi Cola (see soft drinks)	
Perch, fresh	.0 G
Perch, fried with batter, 3 oz.	6.0 G
Persian melon, 1 wedge	12.8 G
Persimmons, 1 medium	20.0 G
Pheasant	.0 G
Pickle relish, 1 T, sw., with additives	3.4 C
Pickle relish, mustard, 1 T sweetened, with additives	3.6 C
Pickles, chow-chow, 4 pieces sw. with additives	1.1 C
Pickles, cucumber, bread and butter, 4 slices, sw. with additives	5.1 C
Pickles, cucumber, 6 sl. sw. with additives	.7 C
Pickles, dill, 1 large	3.0 G
Pickles, sour, 1 large	3.0 G
Pickles, sweet, 1 medium	2.6 C
Pie crust (double crust)	143.0 S
Pie crust, graham cracker (bottom crust)	64.4 C
Pies (all ⅙ of 9" pie, 1 piece)	
Apple	46.7 S
Apricot	57.7 S
Banana cream	35.9 S
Berry	43.0 S
Blackberry	43.0 S
Blueberry	44.0 S
Butterscotch, whipped cream	42.1 S
Cherry	47.7 S
Chocolate chiffon, whipped cream	33.2 S
Chocolate meringue	32.3 S
Coconut custard	30.0 S

Food		Food	
Cream	41.7 S	Pineapple	
Custard	29.9 S	Fresh, 1 C diced	19.0 G
Lemon chiffon	35.2 S	Fresh, 1 slice	11.5 G
Lemon meringue	39.3 S	Canned, 1 large slice w/syrup	26.0 C
Mincemeat	53.9 S	Canned, ½ C crushed	27.5 C
Peach	58.0 S	Canned, low calorie, ½ C	11.0 C
Peach, whipped cream	59.0 S	Candied, 1 slice	30.4 S
Pecan	57.6 S	Frozen, ½ C, sweetened	26.2 C
Pineapple	36.0 S	Pineapple cheese spread (see cheese spreads)	
Pineapple-cheese	38.2 S	Pineapple juice (see juices)	
Pineapple cream	47.5 S	Pistachio nuts, 20	1.6 G
Pizza (see pizza pie)		Pistachio nuts, chopped, 1 T	1.5 G
Prune, whipped cream	53.7 S	Pistachio nuts, shelled, 1 C	24.5 G
Pumpkin	29.4 S	Pizza pie, average piece	25.2 S
Raisin	59.1 S	Plantain, 1	44.3 G
Rhubarb	49.7 S	Plums	
Shoofly	48.3 S	Fresh, 1 medium	7.0 G
Strawberry	51.4 S	Canned, 1 C with syrup	50.0 C
Strawberry cream	53.9 S	Canned, 6 halves with 2 T syrup	25.0 C
Pignolias (see pine nuts)		Canned, low calorie, ½ C	10.0 C
Pig's feet	.0 G	Poha, Hawaiian, 1 C	11.3 G
Pike	.0 G	Polish sausage (see sausage)	
Pimiento, canned, 1 med.	2.2 G	Pomegranate, 1 medium	21.9 G
Pimiento cheese (see cheese)		Pompano	.0 G
Pine nuts, salted, ½ C	5.6 G	Popcorn, no butter, 1 C popped	11.0 G
Pine nuts, chopped, 1 T	.7 G	Popcorn, sugar-coated, 1 oz.	24.1 S

Popover, 1	12.9 S	
Porgy	.0 G	
Pork		
Chops	.0 G	
Heart (see heart)		
Kidney (see kidneys)		
Liver (see liver)		
Pig's feet (see pig's feet)		
Roast	.0 G	
Salt	.0 G	
Sausage (see sausage)		
Shoulder	.0 G	
Sirloin	.0 G	
Spareribs	.0 G	
Tenderloin	.0 G	
Post Toasties (see cereals)		
Postum, 1 t, dry	.8 G	
Pot cheese (see cheese)		
Pot roast (see beef)		
Potato chips, 8 to 10	10.0 S	
Potato salad (see salads)		
Potato soup (see soups)		
Potatoes		
Baked or boiled, 1 med.	21.0 G	
Canned, 3-4 small	19.1 G	
Creamed, ½ C	14.1 G	
French fried, 10 pieces	20.0 C	
French fried, frozen, 10 pieces	15.0 C	
Fried, ½ C	30.9 C	
Hash browned, 1 C	62.2 C	
Mashed, with milk, fresh, ½ C	15.0 G	
Mashed, with milk, butter, fresh, ½ C	14.0 G	
Scalloped, ½ C	14.2 G	
Potatoes, sweet		
Raw, 3½ oz.	27.9 G	
Baked, 1	36.0 G	
Boiled, 1	39.0 G	
Candied, 1 small	60.0 C	
Canned, 1 C	54.0 G	
Dehydrated, 3½ oz.	84.5 G	
Yam, 1 C cooked	48.2 G	
Yam, marshmallow topping, 1 C	60.6 C	
Poultry (see individual listings)		
Poultry stuffing (see stuffing)		
Pound cake (see cakes)		
Preserves (see jams, jellies)		
Pretzels		
Very large, 1	12.7 S	
3 ring, 1	2.4 S	
Sticks, 5 or 1 small	1.4 S	
Prickly pear, 1 med.	4.6 G	
Prosciutto (see ham)		
Protein powders, 1 rounded T	3.0 G	
Prune juice (see juices)		

Prunes		
Medium, 4	19.0	G
Canned, strained, 1 oz.	7.0	G
Cooked, unsw., 1 C with liquid	81.0	G
Cooked, sw. 4-5	31.2	C
Puddings		
Apple brown betty, ½ C	35.2	S
Apple dumpling, 1	54.0	S
Apple snow, ½ C	25.5	S
Banana custard, with meringue, ½ C	19.2	S
Banana whip, ½ C	15.5	S
Bavarian, orange, 1 serving	39.8	S
Blancmange, ½ C	20.0	S
Bread and butter, 1 serving	28.4	S
Bread, with raisins, ¾ C	47.8	S
Butterscotch, ½ C	28.9	S
Butterscotch, sugar-free, ½ C	8.9	S
Caramel, ½ C	28.9	S
Chocolate, ½ C	30.6	S
Chocolate, skim milk, ½ C	30.1	S
Cornstarch, butterscotch, ½ C	37.4	S
Cornstarch, chocolate, ½ C	37.1	S
Cornstarch, vanilla, ½ C	20.0	S
Cottage pudding, 1 piece	43.8	S
Cottage pudding, 2 T lemon sauce, 1 piece	61.1	S
Custard, ½ C	14.0	S
Indian, ⅔ C	22.6	C
Jell-O (see gelatine)	12.2	C
Junket, ½ C	26.5	S
Lemon sponge, 1 serving		
Lemon sponge with custard sauce, 1 serving	41.3	S
Prune whip, ½ C	25.1	C
Rice, with eggs, ½ C	16.8	C
Rice, with raisins, ½ C	32.2	C
Tapioca, ½ C	11.6	C
Tapioca, apricot, ½ C	40.8	C
Tapioca, chocolate, ½ C	32.5	C
Vanilla, ½ C	23.8	C
Pumpkin, 3½ oz.	7.6	G
Pumpkin, canned, 1 C	18.0	G
Pumpkin pie (see pies)		

Q

Quail, broiled	.0	G
Quince, 1 medium	10.2	G
Quinine water (see soft drinks)		

R

Rabbit		
Rabbit stew (see stew)	61.1	S
Radishes, 4 small	14.0	S

Radishes, Chinese, 3½ oz. — 4.5 G
Raisin bread (see breads)
Raisin sauce (see sauces)
Raisins, 1 C — 124.0 G
Raisins, 1 T — 4.5 G
Raisins, 4 — 3.2 G
Raisins, cooked, sw. ½ C — 35.9 C
Ralston (see cereals)
Raspberries
  Black, 1 C — 21.0 G
  Red, 1 C — 17.0 G
Canned, 1 C with syrup — 53.6 C
Canned, water pack, 1 C liquid — 6.2 G
Frozen, 10 oz. carton — 70.0 G
Frozen, 3 oz. — 23.7 G
Raspberry juice (see juices)
Ravioli, cheese filling, 4 squares, sauce — 24.4 C
Red snapper — .0 G
Relish (see pickle relish)
Relish cheese spread (see cheese spreads)
Rhubarb
  Raw, 1 C diced — 4.6 G
  Cooked, sweetened, 1 C — 98.0 C
  Canned, low calorie, 1 C — 4.6 C
  Frozen, ½ C — 22.9 G
Rhubarb pie (see pies)

Rice
Chico San Brown Rice Cracker, 1 — 6.2 G
Brown, 1 C cooked — 43.0 G
Fried, 1 C — 44.0 C
White, 1 C cooked — 44.0 S
White, converted, 1 C cooked — 44.2 S
Wild, 1 C cooked — 30.2 G
Spanish, ¾ C — 26.2 C
Rice Polishings, 2 T — 10.0 G
Rice Krispies (see cereals)
Rice pudding (see puddings)
Rice puffs (see cereals)
Roka bleu cheese spread (see cheese spreads)
Rolls
  Cloverleaf, 1 — 20.5 S
  Hamburger, 1 — 20.9 S
  Hard, 1 large — 31.0 S
  Frankfurter, 1 — 20.5 S
  French, 1 — 20.9 S
  Onion, 1 large — 21.0 S
  Parker House, 1 — 13.5 S
  Plain, 1 — 20.0 S
  Sweet, 1 — 27.0 S
  Whole wheat, 1 — 18.3 G
Romaine, 1 large leaf — .3 G
Roquefort cheese (see cheese)

Rum (see alcohol)	
Russian dressing (see salad dressings)	
Rutabaga, 1 C cooked	11.7 G
Rye bread (see breads)	
Ry-Krisp (see crackers)	

S

Salad dressings

Bacon-vinegar, 1 T	.5 G
Bleu cheese, 1 T	1.2 G
Boiled, home-cooked, 1 T	3.0 G
Commercial, mayonnaise type, 1 T	2.0 G
French, commercial, 1 T	3.0 G
French, homemade, 1 T	2.0 G
Italian, commercial, 1 T	1.0 G
Mayonnaise, 1 T	.4 G
Mayonnaise, with mineral oil, 1 T	.1 S
Roquefort, 1 T	1.2 G
Russian, 1 T	1.5 G
Thousand Island, 1 T	2.2 G
Vinegar and oil, equal parts, 1 T	.4 G

Salads

Apple-carrot, ½ C	11.5 G
Asparagus, 5 spears	3.5 G
Avocado, ½ C with dressing	5.1 G
Avocado-tomato-cottage cheese	9.3 G
Banana and nut, ½ banana	15.2 G
Banana and orange, ½ of each	22.7 G
Carrot-raisin, 3 T	27.9 G
Cole slaw, with French dressing, 1 C	13.6 G
Chicken, with celery, ½ C	2.5 G
Combination vegetable, ½ C	15.8 G
Crab, with celery, ½ C	3.0 G
Egg and tomato, 1 of each	4.3 G
Endive and grapefruit, 1 serving	15.9 G
Fruit, fresh, 3 T	21.2 G
Gelatin, with fruit, 1 square	21.6 C
Gelatin, with vegetables, 1 square	15.1 C
Lettuce and tomatoes	5.8 G
Lettuce with French dressing, 1 wedge	6.9 G
Lobster, with celery, 1 serving	3.0 G
Macaroni, 1 Cup	48.5 S
Mixed greens, with French dressing, ½ C	4.8 G
Orange-grapefruit, with dressing	9.5 G
Potato, with onions, ½ C	13.1 G
Prunes, stuffed with cottage cheese, 4	28.2 G
Salmon, with celery, ½ C	2.5 G
Shrimp, with celery, 1 serving	3.0 G
Tomato and cucumber, 1 of each	8.8 G
Tomato aspic, ½ C	5.4 G
Tuna, with celery, ½ C	2.5 G
Waldorf, ½ C	9.7 G

Salami, 8 oz.	3.0 G	
Salmon		
Broiled or baked	.0 G	
Canned	.0 C	
Creamed, ½ C on toast	16.0 C	
Smoked	.0 G	
Salmon loaf, ½ C	5.1 G	
Salt, table	.0 G	
Sand dabs	.0 G	
Sandwiches	.0 G	
(on whole grain bread only)		
Bacon-egg, 1	24.5 G	
Bacon-tomato-lettuce, 1	28.8 G	
Barbecue beef, 1	24.0 G	
Barbecue pork, 1	24.0 G	
Bologna, 1	25.6 G	
Cervelat, 1	24.0 G	
Cheese, Camembert, 1	24.4 G	
Cheese, Cheddar, 1	26.4 G	
Cheese, Swiss, 1	24.0 G	
Cheese, with olive, 1	25.2 G	
Cheeseburger, 1	22.1 G	
Chicken, sliced, 1	24.0 G	
Chicken liver, 1	25.9 G	
Chicken salad, 1	25.8 G	
Club, 3-decker, 1	41.7 G	
Corned beef, 1	24.0 G	
Crabmeat, 1	25.5 G	
Cream cheese and nut, 1	25.4 G	
Cream cheese and jelly, 1	50.4 C	
Denver, western, 1	27.8 G	
Egg, fried, 1	24.3 G	
Egg salad, 1	24.8 G	
Frankfurter, 1	21.5 G	
Ham, boiled or baked, 1	24.5 G	
Ham, fried, 1	24.0 G	
Ham salad, 1	30.4 G	
Ham and Swiss cheese, 1	25.0 G	
Hamburger, 1	20.9 G	
Liverwurst, 1	24.9 G	
Lobster salad	26.0 G	
Luncheon meat, 1	25.0 G	
Meat loaf, 1	35.9 G	
Oyster, fried, thoroughly cooked, 1	40.7 G	
Pastrami, 1	24.0 G	
Peanut butter, 1	29.3 G	
Peanut butter and jelly, 1	35.3 C	
Pork sausage, 1	24.0 G	
Roast beef, 1	24.0 G	
Roast beef with gravy, 1	27.2 C	
Roast pork, 1	24.0 G	
Roast pork with gravy, 1	27.2 G	
Roquefort spread, 1	25.9 G	
Salami, 1	24.0 G	

Food	Value		Food	Value
Salmon, 1	24.0 G		Custard, 1 T	2.3 C
Salmon salad, 1	25.2 G		Fudge, 1 T	19.0 S
Sardine, 1	24.0 G		Garlic, with butter, 1 T	.5 G
Shrimp, fried, 1 with 6 small	32.2 G		Hard, 1 T	6.0 S
Shrimp salad, 1	26.0 G		Hollandaise, mock, 1/4 C	6.3 G
Sole, fried, 1	36.0 G		Hollandaise, true, 1/4 C	.4 G
Steak, 1	24.0 G		Lemon, 1 T	6.9 C
Tomato and lettuce, 1	26.5 G		Marshmallow, 1 T	6.2 S
Tongue, 1	24.0 G		Meat, Italian, 1 C	20.8 G
Tuna, 1	24.0 G		Mustard, 1/4 C	6.4 G
Tuna salad, 1	25.8 G		Raisin, 1/4 C, sw.	25.9 C
Turkey, 1	24.0 G		Sour cream, 1 T	3.5 G
Turkey with gravy, 1	28.0 C		Soy, 1 T	1.5 G
Vienna sausage, 1	24.0 G		Tartar, 1 T	1.5 G
Sardines			Tomato, 1/4 C	6.0 G
Canned, in oil	.0 G		White, medium, 1/4 C	6.1 S
Canned, in tomato sauce, 1 large	1.0 G		White, thin, 1/4 C	4.6 S
Sauces			Worcestershire, 1 T	2.7 G
A-1, 1 T	2.7 G		Sauerkraut, 1 C drained	7.0 G
Barbecue, 1 T	8.3 S		Sauerkraut juice (see juice)	
Butterscotch, 1 T	20.2 S		Sausage, bologna (see bologna)	
Caramel, 1 T	45.8 S		Sausage, cervelat (see cervelat)	
Cheese, 1/4 C	4.8 G		Sausage, frankfurter (see frankfurter)	
Chili, 1 T	4.0 G		Sausage, liver (see liverwurst)	
Cranberry, 1/4 C, sw.	35.6 C		Sausage, Polish, 4 oz.	1.3 G
Cream, 1 T	1.6 G		Sausage, pork, 8 oz.	trace G
Creole, 1/4 C	7.5 G		Sausage, salami (see salami)	

Sausage, Vienna, canned. 8 oz. — .7 G
Scallions (see onions, green)
Scallops, 2-3 — 3.4 G
Scallops, fried with batter, 3-4 large — 14.6 C
Scampi (see shrimp)
Scotch whisky (see alcohol)
Scrapple, 1 medium slice — 26.0 G
Seafood (see individual listings)
Seafood au gratin, ½ C — 12.1 C
Seltzer water (see soft drinks, soda)
Sesame seeds, 1 oz. — trace G
Shad — .0 G
Sherbets (see ice cream, ices)
Sherry (see alcohol)
Shortbread (see breads)
Shortcake, peach, small serving — 42.4 S
Shortcake, raspberry, medium serving — 47.4 S
Shortcake, strawberry, medium serving — 61.2 S
Shortcake, strawberry sponge medium serving — 60.4 S
Shortening (see butter, Crisco, or lard)
Shredded wheat (see cereals)
Shrimp
Fresh, 7 large or 8 oz. — 2.4 G
Canned, dry pack, 3 oz. — .8 G
Canned, wet pack, 3 oz. — .4 G
Fried, with batter, 3 jumbo — 8.3 C
Scampi, 7 large, in garlic butter — 3.6 G

Shrimp cocktail, with sauce — 7.8 G
Shrimp creole, 7 large, with ½ C sauce — 17.4 G
Smelt — .0 G
Smelt, fried with batter, 2-3 — 10.8 C
Snap beans (see beans, green and wax)
Snow peas, 14-16 — 5.6 G
Sodas (see soft drinks or ice cream sodas)
Sole — .0 G
Soft drinks
Cherry, 8 oz. — 28.0 S
Coca Cola, 8 oz. — 27.0 S
Cream soda, 8 oz. — 28.0 S
Ginger ale, 8 oz. — 21.0 S
Grape, 8 oz. — 28.0 S
Lemon, 8 oz. — 28.0 S
Low calorie, most flavors, 8 oz. — .0 S
Orange, 8 oz. — 28.0 S
Pepsi Cola, 8 oz. — 27.0 S
Root beer, 8 oz. — 28.0 S
Sarsaparilla, 8 oz. — 28.0 S
Soda, seltzer water, 8 oz. — .0 S
Quinine water, 8 oz. — 9.0 S
Soups
(each 1 serving, approx. ¾ C)
Asparagus, cream — 12.5 G
Bean — 18.5 G
Beef noodle — 4.6 G
Beef with vegetable and barley — 7.0 G

Bouillon	.0 G
Celery, cream	12.0 G
Chicken broth	.0 G
Chicken, cream	11.8 G
Chicken, gumbo	12.4 G
Chicken, noodle	6.5 G
Chicken, rice	4.6 G
Chicken, vegetable	7.0 G
Chili beef	18.9 G
Clam chowder, milk	13.5 G
Clam chowder, tomato	8.3 G
Consommé	.0 G
Corn chowder	19.0 G
Green pea	17.5 G
Green pea with ham	14.6 G
Gumbo creole	9.5 G
Jellied consommé	.0 G
Mushroom, cream	13.2 G
Noodle	6.9 G
Onion	3.9 G
Onion, cream	6.8 G
Onion, French	3.9 G
Oyster stew (see oysters)	
Pea, cream	22.6 G
Pepperpot	8.0 G
Potato, cream	13.8 G
Scotch broth	9.1 G
Shrimp, cream	12.0 G
Spinach, cream	11.1 G
Split pea	16.9 G
Tomato, clear	12.0 G
Tomato, cream	14.5 G
Tomato rice	12.7 G
Tomato vegetable	11.0 G
Turkey noodle	7.0 G
Turtle	7.0 G
Vegetable	10.5 G
Vegetable, beef	7.1 G
Vegetable, cream	9.9 G
Vichyssoise	12.2 G
Soybean curd, 1 cake	3.0 G
Soybean milk, ⅜ C	2.1 G
Soybean sprouts, 1 C	10.8 G
Soybeans (see beans)	
Spaghetti	
Cooked, 1 C	44.1 S
Cooked with meat sauce, 1 serving	39.4 C
Cooked, with meatballs	
¾ C, 6 meatballs	43.6 C
Cooked, with tomato sauce	
1 serving	34.3 C
Spareribs (see pork)	
Spices, 1 t	.0 G

Spinach		
Raw, ½ lb.	5.9 G	
Cooked, 1 C	7.2 G	
Canned, 1 C, drained	6.4 G	
Canned, strained, creamed, 1 oz.	2.0 G	
Split pea soup (see soups)		
Spoon bread (see breads)		
Squab	.0 G	
Squash		
Hubbard or winter, baked, ½ C	15.0 G	
Hubbard or winter, frozen boiled, 1 C	9.7	
Summer, boiled, 1 C, drained	7.0 G	
Summer, canned, strained, 1 oz.	1.4 G	
Zucchini, boiled, 1 C, drained	6.3 G	
Squid	.0 G	
Stew		
Beef and vegetable, 1 C	17.0 G	
Lamb and vegetable, 1 C	11.3 G	
Oyster (see oysters)		
Rabbit, 1 C	11.3 G	
Veal and vegetable, 1 C	11.3 G	
Strawberries		
Fresh, 5 large	4.2 G	
Fresh, 1 C	13.0 G	
Frozen, 10 oz. carton	75.0 C	
Frozen, 16 oz. can	100.0 C	
String beans (see beans, green)		

Stroganoff, med. serving	7.0 G	
Stuffing, bread, whole grain, ½ C	28.5 G	
Sturgeon	.0	
Succotash, canned, ½ C	17.6 G	
Succotash, frozen, ½ C	18.9 G	
Sugar		
Beet, ¼ lb.	112.7 S	
Brown, 1 C	210.0 C	
Brown, 1 T	13.0 C	
Confectioner's, 1 C	127.4 S	
Confectioner's, 1 T	8.0 S	
Granulated, 1 C	195.0 S	
Granulated, 1 T	12.0 S	
Granulated, 1 t	4.0 S	
Granulated, 3 cubes	7.0 S	
Granulated, 1 lump	7.0 S	
Maple, 1 inch cube	27.0 C	
Sugar cane juice, 5 T	72.6 G	
Summer squash (see squash)		
Sundaes (see ice cream sundaes)		
Sunflower seeds, 1 T	1.2 G	
Sweet potatoes (see potatoes, sweet)		
Sweetbreads	.0 G	
Sweetbreads, creamed, ½ C	6.1 G	
Swiss chard (see chard)		
Swordfish	.0 G	

Syrups

Item	Value
Chocolate thin-type, 1 T	12.0 S
Chocolate, fudge-type, 1 T	10.5 S
Corn, 1 C	242.0 S
Corn, 1 T	15.0 S
Corn, 1 plastic packet	37.0 S
Honey, 1 T, unrefined	16.4 G
Maple, 1 T	12.8 G
Molasses, light, 1 T	13.0 G
Molasses, medium, 1 T	12.0 G
Molasses, blackstrap, 1 T	11.0 G
Molasses, Barbados, 1 T	14.0 G
Simple sugar, 1 T	7.0 S
Sorghum, 3 oz.	13.4 G
Treacle, 1 T	13.4 G

T

Item	Value
Tangerine juice (see juices)	
Tangerines, 1 medium	10.0 G
Tapioca, ¼ C dry	32.8 C
Tapioca pudding (see puddings)	
Taro, Hawaiian, tubers, 3½ oz.	25.0 G
Taro, Japanese, Dasheen, 3½ oz.	21.2 G
Taro, leaves and stems, 3½ oz.	21.2 G
Tea, 1 C	.4 G
Tea, with 1 T light cream	.9 G
Tea, with 1 T heavy cream	.8 G
Tea, with 1 t lemon	.8 G
Tea, with 1 T milk	1.1 G
Tea, with 1 t sugar	4.4 S
Thousand Island dressing (see salad dressings)	
Toast, bread (see breads, carbohydrate value unchanged)	
Toast, Holland rusk, 1	8.6 S
Toast, Melba, 1 slice	3.9 S
Toast, Zwieback, 1 slice	5.1 C
Tomato catsup (see catsup)	
Tomato juice (see juices)	
Tomato sauce (see sauces)	
Tomato soup (see soups)	
Tomatoes	
Fresh, 1 medium	6.0 G
Fresh, 1 small	4.0 G
Canned, 1 C	9.0 G
Purée, canned, 1 C	18.0 G
Stewed, 1 C	9.0 G
Tongue, beef (see beef)	
Tongue, canned, 3 medium slices	.2 G
Tortilla, 1 5"	4.5 C
Tripe, boiled	.0 G
Tripe, pickled	.0 G
Trout, brook	.0 G
Trout, lake	.0 G

Tuna
  Fresh or canned .0 G
  Casserole, with noodles, 1 serving 25.0 C
Turkey
  Roasted or smoked .0 G
  Creamed, 4 oz. 6.1 G
  Pot pie, frozen, 8 oz. 50.4 C
  Potted .0 G
Turkey hash (see hash)
Turnip greens, 1 C cooked 8.0 G
Turnip greens, canned, 1 C 7.0 G
Turnips, 1 C diced 9.0 G
Turnips, cooked, 1 4.7 G
Turtle .0 G

V

Vanilla extract, 1 t .1 G
Vanilla ice cream (see ice cream)
Vanilla pudding (see puddings)
Veal
  Chop .0 G
  Cutlet .0 G
  Cutlet, breaded, 1 med. 16.0 G
  Kidney (see kidneys)
  Roast .0 G
  Stew (see stew)
  Stewing meat
Veal Goulash (see goulash, Hungarian)
Vegetable juice (see juices)
Vegetable and meat stew (see stew)
Vegetable soup (see soups)
Vegetables (see individual listings)
Vegetables, mixed, canned, 4 oz. 15.1 G
Vegetables, mixed, frozen, 4 oz. 15.7 G
Venison .0 G
Vienna sausage (see sausage)
Vinegar, 1 T .8 G

W

Waffles, 1 medium 30.0 S
Walnuts, black, 1 C chopped 19.0 G
Walnuts, black, 8-10 halves 2.8 G
Walnuts, English, 8-16 halves 2.3 G
Walnuts, English, 1 C chopped 17.6 G
Walnuts, English, 1 T chopped 1.0 G
Water chestnuts, 4 4.5 G
Water cress (see cress)
Watermelon, 1 slice, 1½"x6" 38.4 G
Watermelon, 1 wedge, 1/16 of melon 57.6 G
Watermelon, balls or cubes, ½ C 6.9 G
Wax beans (see beans)
Welsh rabbit, medium serving, on toast 23.5 G

Wheat germ, 1 T	3.7 G
Whipped cream (see cream)	
White fish, steamed or smoked	.0 G
White fish, baked, stuffed, 1 serving	
White sauce (see sauces)	11.6 G
Wine (see alcohol)	

Y

Yams (see potatoes, sweet)	
Yeast, 1 cake	3.7 C
Yeast, brewer's, 1 rounded T	3.0 G
Yeast, brewer's, tablets, 10	1.4 G
Yogurt, skim milk, 1 C	11.7 G

Z

Zucchini (see squash)	
Zwiebach (see toast)	

Alcoholic Beverages

Beers, ciders	
Ale, light, 8 oz.	8.0 S
Ale, imported, 8 oz.	10.0 S
Beer, 8 oz.	11.0 S
Cider, fermented, 6 oz.	1.8 C
Porter or stout, 8 oz.	10.0 S

Cocktails, highballs (1)	
Alexander, brandy	4.0 S
Bacardi cocktail	3.3 S
Bloody Mary	5.1 S
Bourbon highball, soda	.0 S
Bourbon highball, ginger ale	15.7 S
Champagne cocktail	9.0 S
Daiquiri	5.2 S
Eggnog	18.0 S
Gimlet	1.2 S
Gin and tonic, 10 oz.	9.0 S
Gin rickey	1.3 S
Grasshopper	18.0 S
Hot buttered rum	trace S
Irish coffee	5.5 C
Manhattan	7.9 S
Martini	.3 S
Mint julep	2.7 S
Old Fashioned	3.5 S
Orange blossom	3.7 S
Pink lady	3.0 S
Planter's punch	7.9 S
Rob Roy, with dry vermouth	.1 S
Rum and cola	20.4 S
Rum punch	7.9 S
Rye highball, ginger ale	15.7 S
Rye highball, soda	.0 S

Sazarac	2.5 S
Scotch highball, soda	.0 S
Scotch mist	.0 S
Screwdriver	15.0 S
Sidecar	4.2 S
Sloe gin fizz	1.3 S
Stinger	9.0 S
Tom Collins	9.0 S
Whiskey sour	3.9 S
Liquors, whiskeys	
Bourbon whiskey, 1½ oz.	.0 S
Canadian whiskey, 1½ oz.	.0 S
Gin, 1½ oz.	.0 S
Irish whiskey, 1½ oz.	.0 S
Rum, 1½ oz.	.0 S
Rye whiskey, 1½ oz.	.0 S
Scotch whiskey, 1½ oz.	.0 S
Sloe gin, 1½ oz.	.0 S
Vodka, 1½ oz.	.0 S
Liqueurs, brandies	
Anisette, 1 oz.	7.0 S
Applejack, 1 oz.	trace S
Benedictine, 1 oz.	6.6 S
Brandy, 1 oz.	.0 S
Chartreuse, 1 oz.	6.6 S
Cherry Heering, 1 oz.	6.0 S
Crème de Cacao, 1 oz.	6.0 S
Crème de menthe, 1 oz.	6.0 S
Curacao, 1 oz.	6.0 S
Kummel, 1 oz.	6.0 S
Wines	
Champagne, dry, domestic, 4 oz.	3.0 G
Champagne, dry, French, 4 oz.	1.0 G
Dinner, dry red—Chianti, Claret, Burgundy, 3½ oz.	.5 G
Dinner, dry white—Chablis, Moselle, Rhine, 3½ oz.	.5 G
Dinner, Sauterne, 3½ oz.	4.0 G
Dubonnet, 3 oz.	12.0 S
Madeira, 3½ oz.	3.0 G
Malaga, 3½ oz.	20.0 S
Muscatel, 3½ oz.	14.0 S
Port, 3½ oz.	14.0 S
Sherry, 3½ oz.	4.8 C
Vermouth, dry, 3½ oz.	1.0 G
Vermouth, sweet, 3½ oz.	12.0 S

Suggested Reading

The following books will give you more information about nutrition and health. They are available in health stores, or book stores can order them for you.

		Publisher
Linda Clark:		
STAY YOUNG LONGER	Paperback	Pyramid
GET WELL NATURALLY	Paperback	Arco
SECRETS OF HEALTH AND BEAUTY	Paperback	Pyramid
FACTS ABOUT FACE EXERCISES	Paperback	Keats
Adelle Davis:		
LET'S EAT RIGHT TO KEEP FIT	Paperback	Signet
LET'S HAVE HEALTHY CHILDREN	Paperback	Signet
LET'S GET WELL	Hardback	Harcourt Brace & World
Catharyn Elwood:		
FEEL LIKE A MILLION	Paperback	Pocket Books
Carlton Fredericks (with Herman Goodman, M.D.):		
LOW BLOOD SUGAR AND YOU	Hardback	Constellation
Beatrice Trum Hunter:		
FACT/BOOK ON ADDITIVES	Paperback	Keats
Carlson Wade		
FACT/BOOK ON VITAMINS AND OTHER FOOD SUPPLEMENTS	Paperback	Keats

Cook Books (which show how to use the high powered foods in cooking):

Adelle Davis:		
LET'S COOK IT RIGHT	Paperback	Signet
Beatrice Trum Hunter:		
THE NATURAL FOODS COOK BOOK	Paperback	Pyramid
Gena Larson:		
FACT/BOOK ON BETTER FOOD FOR BETTER BABIES	Paperback	Keats
Agnes Toms:		
EAT, DRINK AND BE HEALTHY	Paperback	Pyramid

Due to my heavy schedule, I regret that I cannot correspond with readers. The above books will answer most of your questions. I do report research and answer general questions in a column, "Light on Your Problems," which appears monthly in *Let's LIVE* magazine, 444 North Larchmont Blvd., Los Angeles, Ca. 90004.